The Emergence of Helicopters and Hospitals

From Vietnam to Hospital Air Ambulances

Eileen Frazer, RN

The Emergence of Helicopters and Hospitals
From Vietnam to Hospital Air Ambulances

by Eileen Frazer, RN

KDP/Amazon Edition

paperback: ISBN: 979-8-9861971-0-4

Library of Congress Control Number: TXu2-325-027

685 Spring Street, PMB #140 Friday Harbor, WA 98250
Contact: eileen.frazer0520@gmail.com

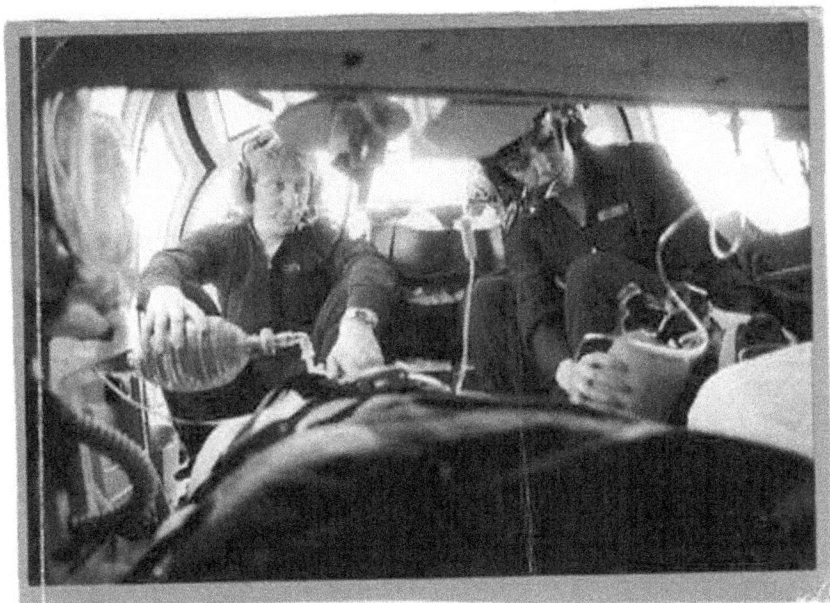

Eileen Frazer, RN, and Rick Shurgalla, paramedic, caring for
two trauma patients in a BO105 helicopter in 1988.

Our lives as we lead them as passed on to others, whether in physical or mental forms, tingeing all future lives together. This should be enough for one who lives for truth and service to his fellow passengers on the way.
—Luther Burbank

PROLOGUE

It was 1985. He sat quietly off to one side of the room, contributing but not dominating the conversations. I was Chair of a new Air Medical Safety Committee, and we were attempting to understand what was needed to lower the number of recent civilian helicopter accidents while transporting patients and medical teams.

The helicopter was brought into the civilian landscape by hospital trauma centers in the 1970s and 1980s. The growth of these services has never stopped and because of helicopter air ambulances, most Americans with severe injuries or critical illnesses are within a few minutes of a major medical center.

The Korean War experience of transporting 20,000 wounded was surpassed by the Vietnam War where 900,000 wounded were transported to battlefield surgical units lowering the mortality rate to one per 100 casualties.[1] The lessons learned were transposed to civilian life in the U.S. as public and financial support for Trauma Centers emphasized the need for helicopter services.

Major hospitals borrowed the military experiences to support the development of trauma centers and to contract with aviation operators for helicopters, pilots, and maintenance. Pilots hired for these services were mostly surviving Vietnam pilots (where the life expectancy of a helicopter pilot was between 13 and 30 days).[2] But we were not in a combat zone. On the clinical side, nurses and paramedics were accustomed to the hospital and EMS environment but not familiar with aviation, especially with helicopters, so the two disciplines were coming from quite different backgrounds and experiences.

Trying to write safety guidelines for pilots who still had "completing the mission" as their goal and nurses and paramedics who were newly exposed to aviation was our challenge. In chairing the committee, I did not know it at the time, but that "quiet man" was an officer in Air America before the Vietnam War and piloted one of the last civilian flights out of Da Nang in 1975.

History, aviation, and medicine are my passion. In my professional career, I have been fortunate to meet and work with leaders who have developed the civilian medical transport systems in the U.S. These helicopter air ambulance (HAA) services have saved countless lives and continue to impact healthcare delivery in urban and rural communities.

These are personal accounts of how the Vietnam experiences influenced the development of trauma centers through the memories of three key influencers at a time when helicopter manufacturers were looking for a new marketplace.

—Eileen Frazer, RN

Sources: 1.) http://www.militaryfactory.com/vietnam/caualties.php

2.) http://sovnow.com/index.php?/news/article/vietnam_dustoff_pilots/

The Emergence of Helicopters and Hospitals

Table of Contents

Chapter One

My Role with Civilian Helicopter Air Ambulance Development in the U. S.

A friend asked me recently: "Why did you want to write this book?" After forty years in this profession, my quick answer was, "I feel so fortunate to have met some wonderful, bright and inspiring people along my journey." I did not want to make this autobiographical, but we all live in the context of our experiences, and I have lived in this time and space for the last forty years. As a perpetual student of American history, I wanted to relate the historical intersection of aviation, medicine, and business development that I chronicle through the individual human experiences that are integral to this history.

My personal journey and involvement with helicopters and medicine began in 1980. I was a part-time night nurse in the Emergency Department (ED) at a Level I Trauma Center in Allentown, PA. I had a young daughter and wanted to spend as much time with her as possible, so night shift allowed me to be with her every day – sharing naps and Sesame Street. That summer our head nurse, Ms. Creamer, died after a painful struggle with pancreatic cancer. Soon after her memorial service, I was summoned to the Director of Nursing's office. I had only met Ms. Vaugh personally one time and that was at Ms. Creamer's memorial service.

I had no idea why Ms. Vaughn wanted to see me but soon learned that, before she died, Ms. Creamer asked that I be named her replacement as head nurse. I had a lot of admiration for Ms. Creamer, and she was well-respected by the physicians and nurses, but this was totally unexpected. After discussing this new job opportunity with my husband and daughter and clearing after-school arrangements, I accepted the position. I had no experience as a nurse manager, but I had thirteen years' experience in the ED, and I felt like I could do it. Growing up as the oldest of five siblings provides a depth of leadership experience and I was up for the challenge. Of course, this would never happen in today's environment. I graduated from a three-year nursing school. I had college credits but not a degree and certainly was never a manager. But suddenly I found myself in charge of seventy employees in a busy Level I trauma center emergency department. I look back on this as sort of destiny because without this happening I would not have been in position for my next chapter.

In 1981, our Chief of Trauma, Dr. Michael Rhodes, who did his Acute Care Surgery fellowship with Dr. Cowley in Baltimore, petitioned the hospital to start a hospital-based helicopter program. It made sense because Allentown is surrounded by major highways and rural farmlands. Philadelphia is 60 miles south and New York City 90 miles east as the next largest centers for trauma at that time.

Dr. Rhodes started a training program for nurses in the ED who wanted to be assigned as a flight nurse when the program started. I was hooked and trained right along with twenty of my staff in the OR for endotracheal intubations. We completed the Advanced Trauma Life Support (ATLS) and paramedic courses in the six months prior to starting the actual helicopter service in May of 1981. Interestingly, one of the ED nurses, Carol Bury, was put in charge of scheduling the training, but she wanted nothing to do with flying in a helicopter. Between Carol and me, we decided to ask the Director of Nursing if we could switch roles. Carol wanted the head nurse position, and I loved the challenge of this new nursing role. That was all we had to do, and suddenly Carol was the ED Head Nurse, and I was a Chief Flight Nurse. Again – an unprecedented move by management. There was really no job description or qualifications on paper for my new position, so we made it up as we developed. As I reached out to several other programs, many of the Chief Flight Nurses were as inexperienced as I was in this new and rapidly growing air ambulance profession.

In 1981, we were the 17th hospital-based helicopter program to develop in the U.S. By July 1990, there were 174 hospital-based helicopter programs. Table 1 (next page) provides a summary of the number of programs and how they were increasing each year as well as helicopter makes, models, manufacturers and names of the aviation operators who were contracting with hospitals at that time. There are 12 aviation operators in this chart. Today only three of those operators remain active in air medicine: Air Methods, Metro Aviation, and Petroleum Helicopters (rebranded as PHI Air Medical). Another major operator, Global Medical Response (GMR) has several entities covering a large percentage of programs in the U.S. today. The other previous operators either merged or went out of the air ambulance business.

When I refer to a "program" I am referring to the helicopter service, usually with a specific identifier such as "Life Flight" or "Medevac" that is familiar to many who live in populated communities. Most of the 17 nurses in my position at newly developed programs during that time had similar backgrounds as emergency department or critical care nurse managers but few had flight nursing experience.

My First Flight

I think my first flight illustrates exactly what I did not know and what most nurses entering this field today would not believe. I was on night duty on Friday, May 5, 1981 when we received our first request for an interfacility transport of a trauma patient from a small rural hospital – about a 10-minute flight. The surgical resident joined me, and we waited on the helipad for the helicopter to arrive from Keystone Helicopters – located in West Chester to the South. The hospital had not formally contracted with the aviation operator to have a helicopter standing by at the hospital. This entire idea was still in trial mode. As we stood there – I realized I had never been in a helicopter and had never even been close enough to look inside. I expressed my concern to the resident, and he said not to worry – he had been in Vietnam, and he knew all about helicopters.

When the pilot landed, the resident warned me to stay back – which I kind of knew from watching MASH. The pilot shut down

My Role With CIvilian Helicopter Air Ambulance Development in the U. S.

Table 1

HOSPITAL-BASED HELICOPTERS

July 1, 1990

General	July 1985	July 1986	July 1987	July 1988	July 1989	July 1990
Programs	101	129	145	155	165	174
Cities	85	111	125	131	136	137
Helicopters	119	151	184	195	213	231
Operators	34	37	31	33	32	27
Patients (000)	60	78	93	104	111	119
Helicopters - single turbine						
LongRanger	31	36	42	45	42	43
AStar	17	25	23	25	19	22
Alouette	9	10	11	8	6	5
JetRanger	5	5	3	0	2	0
Other	2	2	0	0	0	0
Subtotal	**64**	**78**	**79**	**78**	**69**	**70**
Helicopters - twin turbine						
BK-117	7	16	31	44	55	59
BO-105	17	16	21	25	34	36
TwinStar	16	17	17	13	13	12
Dauphin 365	1	3	9	12	15	14
Bell 222	8	13	14	9	9	11
Agusta 109	6	7	9	9	7	8
Sikorsky S76	0	0	3	5	7	12
Bell 212/412	0	0	0	3	4	9
Sikorsky 58T	0	1	1	1	0	0
Subtotal	**55**	**73**	**105**	**121**	**144**	**161**
% Twins	46%	48%	57%	61%	68%	70%
Manufacturer						
W German	20%	21%	28%	35%	42%	41%
American	38%	37%	34%	31%	30%	32%
French	37%	37%	33%	29%	25%	23%
Italian	5%	5%	5%	5%	3%	3%
Operator contracts						
Rocky Mountain	21	31	35	38	42	43
Omniflight	15	15	18	21	22	40
Air Methods	5	7	8	9	9	12
Corporate Jets	unk	unk	unk	unk	unk	11
Petroleum	2	2	4	8	9	9
St. Louis	4	4	5	5	6	6
Metro Aviation	2	4	4	5	6	6
Keystone	1	2	3	4	5	5
Indianapolis Heliport	unk	unk	unk	unk	unk	4
Hospital AirTransport	3	2	4	3	4	3
SilverStar	4	8	10	16	15	(A)
US Jet	2	5	6	7	10	(B)
Other*	22	25	19	23	22	18
Hospital**	8	11	17	13	14	16
Services						
Shared	18%	16%	17%	15%	14%	unk
Competing	31%	42%	40%	46%	49%	unk

*Ranked according to 1990 data (A) Merged with Omniflight
**Operators with two or less contracts (B) Merged with Corporate Jets
***Hospitals with own flight department

1985-1990 List of Helicopters, Manufacturers and Operators

and got out to open the doors and help us get settled and belted in our seats. We were told to put headsets on and how to press and talk. We lifted off, and as we continued North, the pilot seemed to have lost some lights in the cockpit. He was shining a flashlight, which he held in his teeth, to see the instruments. I thought this was odd, but what did I know?

The pilot told us he had just practiced landing at this hospital and others in the area, so he was familiar with the parking lot they had roped off for helicopter landings. What the pilot did not know was that at midnight, all the parking lot lights were switched off to save on power. He had to radio back to the trauma center and ask them to call the hospital to turn on the parking lot lights. Apparently, the ED had not coordinated the request for the helicopter with their security people.

As we circled, the lights finally came on. We landed and the pilot told us to stay seated until he shut down. When we exited, he showed us how to retrieve the stretcher. This was a Messer-schmitt-Bolkow-Blohm (MBB) BO105 helicopter and fortunately the ED staff was waiting with one of their wheeled gurneys to put our stretcher and supplies on.

The patient was an 18-year-old motor vehicle accident victim. He was unresponsive. We had to intubate and stabilize fractures of the left arm and left leg. The resident suspected internal injuries and said we had better hurry. We secured him to our stretcher and moved him over to the ED gurney and wheeled him out to the helicopter.

Up to this point, we thought we were doing pretty good but when we went to put him head-first into the tunnel of the BO105, the pilot said: "It cannot go in that way!" We did not realize there was a head and foot section to the stretcher, and we had the patient on upside down. We could not possibly leave him on with his head and chest stuck back in the tunnel, so we had no choice. We took him out and went back to the ED to take him off the stretcher, turn it around and move him again to put his head where it needed to be. I was thankful he did not appear to be aware of the pain we caused by moving him on and off the stretcher.

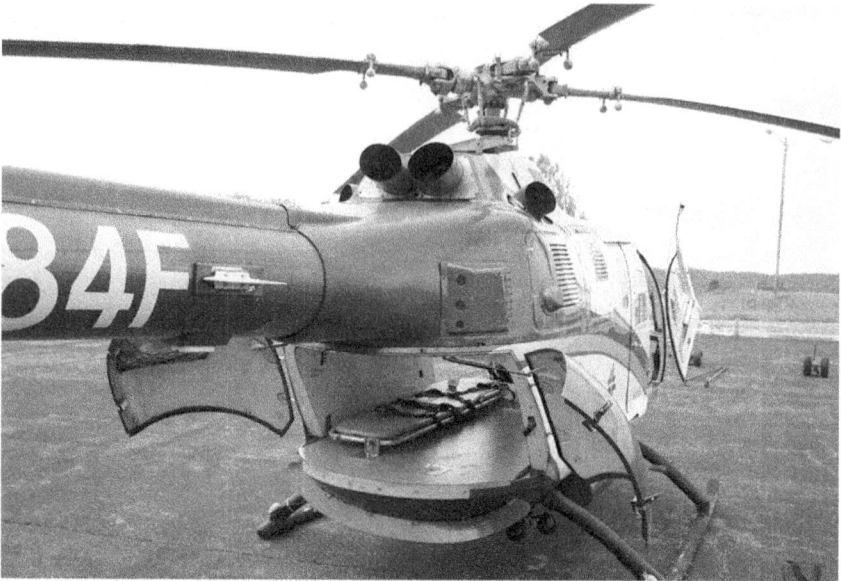

A picture of a BO105 depicting the open clam shell doors where the patient is slid into the aircraft

The patient did not deteriorate during the short flight and when we landed at the trauma center, the entire 7 floors of windows facing the helipad were filled with staff clapping and smiling, celebrating the first flight.

The head trauma physician, Dr. Rhodes, was on duty. He was also smiling, and he never smiles. He asked me why I looked upset. I asked him to come back and see me after he was done in surgery, and I would explain.

Around 4:00 AM, the trauma surgeon came to my office, where I was already writing some notes about what I should have known, and what I learned from this humiliating experience. We discussed it and he agreed we would not accept another request until we had all the nurses and residents become familiar with the helicopter: how to open and close doors, rules about seat belts, how to properly secure and load the patient, how the headsets worked and what emergencies we might encounter and how to handle them. I still wonder why we had not thought to include this in all the training we did up until that first flight – but we were focused on the patient – not the unfamiliar environment.

The helicopter showed up the next afternoon, giving me time to call staff in and put together a "need to know" orientation and checklist. This was only the beginning.[2]

Surviving a Fatal Accident

I began to reach out to search for practice standards for civilian flight crews and only found military protocols which did not mimic our practice of inter-hospital and scene transports in small helicopters. In 1982, I experienced first-hand that we knew little about what was needed to provide safe transport for the patients and crews.

It was a dark and rainy night on April 27 when we received a request for an auto accident victim about 20 miles west of Allentown. Prior to accepting the flight request, the pilot checked the weather reports, and the ceiling and visibility were not below our weather minimums.

The flight crew responded and landed in an open field where a landing site had been set up by EMS and Fire personnel, who helped to load the patient into the helicopter. At midnight, our helicopter was departing the scene with a very combative young male patient. They were in the air less than a minute when they crashed, killing all four on board.

The NTSB listed the causes as:

#1: LOSS OF CONTROL - IN FLIGHT Phase of Operation: CRUISE Findings

1. (F) LIGHT CONDITION - DARK NIGHT

2. (F) WEATHER CONDITION - LOW CEILING

3. (F) WEATHER CONDITION - RAIN

4. (F) IN-FLIGHT PLANNING/DECISION- IMPROPER - PILOT IN COMMAND.

Weather reports at that time required phoning the Flight Service Station to get the most current weather briefing and forecast. There was no internet and no instant weather reporting like there is today.

The pilot, Jimmy, was the Lead Pilot's best friend. The nurse, Jeannette, was my classmate from nursing school. The paramedic, Patty, was quite young and had switched shifts with one of the other paramedics for that night. She was not originally scheduled - which her mother reminded me at the funeral. The patient was an eighteen-year-old male – big and strong, and according to EMS ground services, inebriated and combative.

The aircraft they were in was the same MBB BO 105 when I described my first flight. The stretcher slid in from the rear with the patient's head and chest ending up at the feet of the paramedic who was facing aft and sitting next to the pilot. The nurse sat on the side seat – all small and compact quarters. Although the NTSB found this was a weather-related accident, they had only been in the air a few seconds after lift-off from the scene before they crashed. We felt certain the patient had become more combative. He may have pushed the paramedic into the pilot and into the controls which were unprotected (no barrier) since they came down in a hard right turn.

The accident brought the Lead Pilot, Rick Frazer (who became my second husband and life partner) and me together in our common desire to prevent this tragedy from happening to others. We learned so much from this accident including how the community felt about Medevac. The outpouring of sympathy and kindness from the community was unbelievable. The support from the local EMS also made us realize how much we depended on EMS and Fire departments and how much we appreciated each other's role in saving lives at the risk of possibly losing our own.

When word got around about the fatal accident that night, EMS, and off-duty personnel from all around the area in Eastern PA showed up at the hospital. We set up conference rooms for the families and I sat with them while we waited to hear about their loved ones' remains and conditions at the site. I had met Jeannette's husband and two sons in the past and they were anxious to talk to me. We all handle shock and grief differently and I was expecting some outrage or anger, but I was surprised at what they told me. The older son looked at me and said, "Please don't let my mom die in vain."

I asked him what he meant, and he told me how much she loved being a flight nurse and how she felt about taking care of patients who may have died in the past due to lengthy ground transports. Listening to him, I could hear Jeanette's excitement and enthusiasm about her role as a flight nurse. Her son hoped this accident and her death would not be responsible for causing the hospital to close the program.

There were several physicians and administrators on the hospital staff who felt that was just what should happen. They expressed that this was too much of a risk. But Dr. Rhodes kept stressing how important the helicopter was to the hospital and its new designation as a Level I Trauma Center. We attended a meeting with the CEO and Board of Directors and after some hesitation, they decided to keep going and we did. We went out of service for only one week while Keystone Helicopters configured a replacement helicopter (a Bell 206). But we still had a lot to learn.

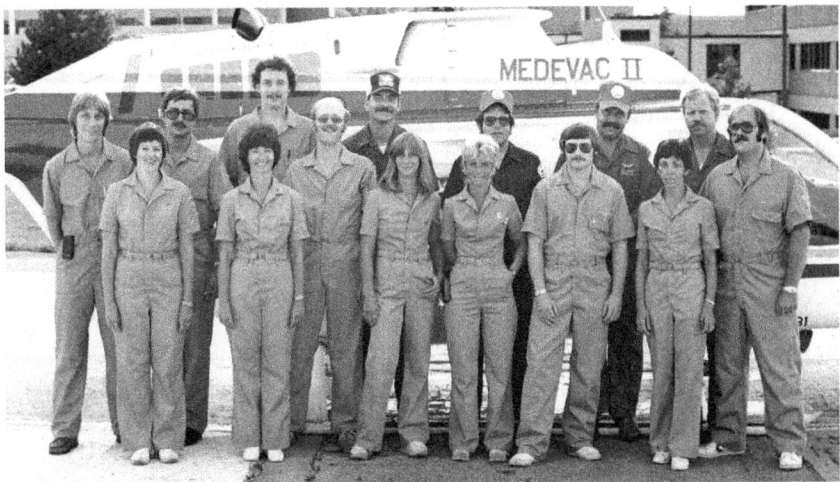

Medevac – replacement Bell Long Ranger

Changes to address future challenges

When the accident occurred, we did not have a policy that the crew should decide to transport the patient by ground if too combative. We did not have a policy for Rapid Sequence Intubation (RSI) at the time. This technique paralyzes a patient who needs an airway and allows the provider to intubate, and it is also a form of chemical restraint. In the early 1980s we only had physical restraints and we would tie the patient's hands and feet to the stretcher. There were no barriers in any air medical aircraft at the time to protect the pilot and controls from patient or crew interference. In a BO105 helicopter, the pilot and controls are within arm's reach of the crew member, who is facing aft, in the seat next to him. When the stretcher is slid in and locked, the patient's head is at the feet of the that crew member.

We did not anticipate all these hazards. That became obvious *after* the accident, but we made immediate changes where we could. We petitioned the helicopter manufacturers, especially MBB and Bell Helicopters. These were small helicopters primarily used for air medical transport, where the patient could potentially encounter the pilot and controls, either by reaching his arms (in the BO105) or kicking with his legs (in the Bell Long Ranger). We knew the aircraft had to undergo a Supplemental Type Certification (FAA - STC) to configure a permanent barrier, and that cost money and time. But, after this accident, we published and spoke at conferences to encourage that a barrier be installed in these helicopters to physically protect the pilot and controls from unintended interference by the patient or crew.

In the 1980s, we experienced rapid expansion with more and more hospital-based helicopter services opening across the U.S. The accident rate increased exponentially with 15 fatal helicopter accidents and 22 deaths in 1986. Rick and I traveled to the National Transportation Safety Board (NTSB) in DC on a quarterly basis, looking through endless microfiche files to collect EMS helicopter accident reports. At the time these were not digital files, and they were not categorized as EMS accidents, so we had to review all the reports to determine which accident involved transporting a patient.

FIGURE 5

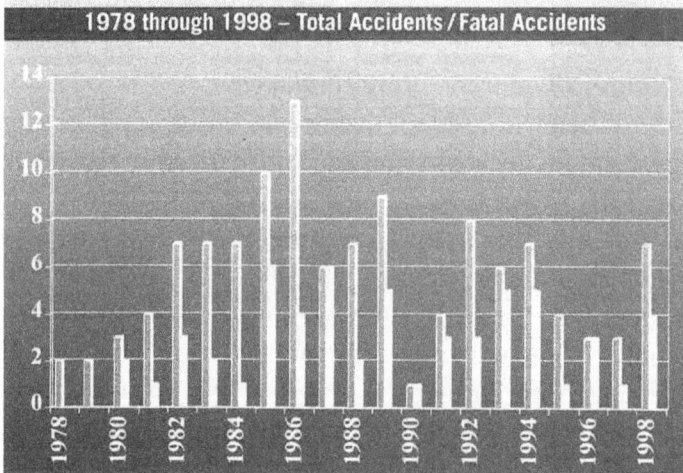

1978 through 1998 – Total Accidents / Fatal Accidents

(Total accidents are represented by the gray bar. The white bar represents the number of those accidents in that year that had at least 1 fatality)

We built an extensive data base, published findings, and lectured at conferences throughout the 1980s and 1990s. In the twenty-year span between 1978 to 1998, there was a total of 122 total accidents in our database, but final reports from the NTSB are usually two to three years behind and we did not enter data that was not verifiable by the NTSB reports. There were NTSB final reports for 107 accidents (as depicted in the Figure 5 bar graph on p.18). In those accident reports, we studied things like total versus fatal accidents (meaning there was at least 1 fatality on board), interfacility versus scene, and phase of flight in which the accident occurred.

Takeoffs and landings are recognized as the most critical phases of flight, but our data showed that more accidents occurred during cruise than in takeoffs and landings combined. (Phase of Flight and Rotorwing Accidents by Cause charts - current page - as referenced in Rick Frazer's 1999 study "Air medical accidents - a 20-year search for information").[3]

This made sense when we looked at causes as determined by the NTSB. Most of the cruise

Air Medical Accidents by Phase of Flight

	Rotor-wing	Fixed-wing
Approach	10	7
Climb	2	0
Cruise	39	2
Descent	3	2
Hover	6	0
Landing	10	1
Maneuvering	9	0
Takeoff	28	2
Taxiing	0	1

Rotor-wing Accidents by Cause

	Total number	Fatal accidents
PILOT		
Weather	23	17
Spatial disorientation	5	4
Hit obstacle	19	3
Hover	3	1
Takeoff	10	2
Low level cruise	2	2
Landing	3	1
Loss of control	12	3
High rate of descent	4	0
Tail rotor authority	2	0
Low downwind turn	4	2
Other	2	1
Fuel starvation	2	2
Other	2	0
Foreign object into a/c	3	0
Engine: wrong shutdown	2	2
IFR: failure to follow	1	1
MECHANICAL		
Engine	14	2
Single	10	
Twin	4	
Flight controls	8	3
Improper maintenance	4	0
UNKNOWN	3	0
TO BE DETERMINED	9	5

(Totals are calculated from NTSB data 1978-1998)

accidents were weather related and occurred at night, a cause that is common to helicopters and fortunately occur with less frequency in today's environment of advanced technology, instruments, risk assessment tools, and weather reporting.

Technologies and Practices Available and Widely Used for HAA Today Versus the Previous Decade. [7]

	1994- 2003	2004-present
Night Vision Goggles	No	Yes
Satellite Tracking	No	Yes
GPS mapping Software	No	Yes
HTAWS	No	Yes
CRM/AMRM	No	Yes
Safety Management System	No	Yes
Operational Control	No	Yes
Flight Simulators	No	Yes
Hospital instrument approaches	No	Yes
Improved weather reporting	No	Yes

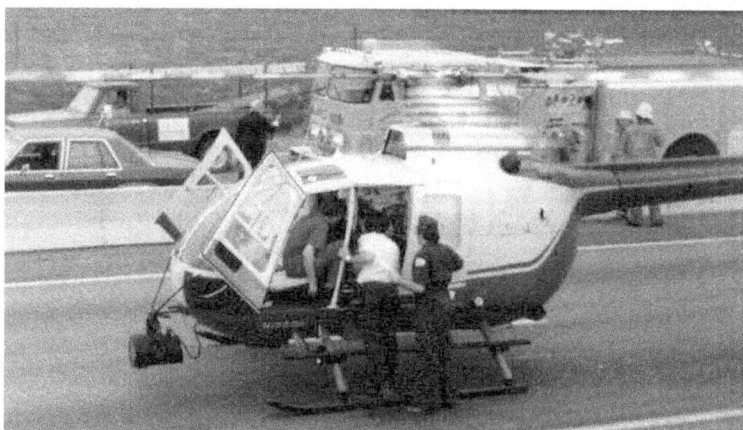

Before there was wide use of NVGs, pilots depended on a huge spotlight off the nose of the aircraft called a Night Sun for night scene landings as seen in this 1986 picture on a PA highway

In 1985, I became Chair of the Air Medical Safety Committee for American Society of Hospital-Based Emergency Air Medical Services (ASHBEAMS) now branded as the Association of Air Medical Services (AAMS) and we were determined to make representation multidisciplined from all corners of the country. We had nurses, paramedics, communicators, and pilots volunteering to serve on the committee. By 1986, accidents were increasing at an alarming rate, and we knew we needed efforts from all disciplines to address findings in the NTSB accident files. We started by comparing policies and safety practices that we could share and develop into guidelines. There were no standards at the time. Hospitals were accustomed to developing patient care protocols but those did not address common practices that could be unsafe for the crew and/or patient during transport. For example, when CPR is started - it is to be continued without interruptions until the patient responds or is pronounced dead by a physician. However, during the critical phases of flight (takeoffs and landings) everyone must be belted into their seats – an FAA regulation. In most aircraft, this is not possible to do and still reach the patient's chest to perform chest compressions. Therefore, CPR must be discontinued until in level flight or after landing.

The Safety Committee conducted a survey regarding common practices which resulted in a study that was published in 1987. This study compared things like: responsibilities of medical crew related to flight operations, medical crew fitness standards, rest/sleep policies and education topics included in training medical personnel. Aviation topics for medical personnel were stressed through various conferences and publications in the previous few years and we found that some of these topics were at least part of medical crews' orientation and annual training, according to our data. This study allowed the Safety Committee to see where we needed to provide more emphasis going forward.[4]

The total number that responded to the questionnaire was 113 (about 87% of the programs at that time). Answering 0 under the "No" heading means there was no one trained in that topic.

Components of Medical Crew Education and Training						
			Response Frequencies (as % of total)			
Topics	n	No	Orient Only	Annual	Semi- Annual	Bi- Annual	Other
Air Physiology	111	3.6	37.8	33.4	0.9	0	24.3
Aircraft familiarization	113	0	15.0	44.2	8.0	1.8	31.0
Safety in & around aircraft	113	0	5.3	47.6	10.6	1.8	32.7
Emergency egress	112	2.7	9.8	47.3	8.9	2.7	28.6
Emergency landing procedures	113	1.8	9.7	48.6	8.0	1.8	30.1
Aircraft fuel shut-down	113	12.6	8.0	43.7	8.0	1.8	25.9
Radio operations	113	2.7	13.2	42.5	8.0	0.9	32.7
Emergency frequencies	113	7.1	12.4	44.2	7.1	0.9	28.3
ELT location/operation	113	10.6	12.4	46.0	6.2	0.9	23.9
Loran location/operation	113	38.1	13.3	27.4	4.4	0	16.8
Aircraft power shut-down	112	14.3	9.8	41.1	7.1	1.8	25.9
Survival training	111	23.4	12.6	38.8	4.5	0	20.7
Water rescue/survival	113	62.8	6.2	16.8	1.8	1.8	10.6

Association of Air Medical Services (AAMS) Study in 1986

Training for crews was just one issue and we looked for trends and tried to learn from each new NTSB final report. Rick and I continued to visit the NTSB in the 1980s as we were developing safety guidelines for the Association of Air Medical Services (formerly ASHBEAMS). The National Transportation Safety Board continued to research HEMS causes and raise awareness. The high rate of fatal accidents in 1986 led to a study by NTSB's Robert Dodd, PhD, that was published in 1988.[5] This study evaluated 59 HEMS accidents and found that the accident rate was nearly double that of other FAA Part 135 operations and the fatal accident rate was nearly 3.5 times other Part 135 Operations. This study also resulted in 19 safety recommendations to the FAA and air medical transport services, and these recommendations were part of the draft in the first edition of accreditation standards for the new organization that was incorporated in 1990.

Development of accreditation

In 1987, the President of ASHBEAMS, Jim Smith, where I served on the Board as Chair of the Air Medical Safety Committee, promised the members that we would develop Priority One – a peer review safety audit. Our committee quickly developed guidelines for Priority One to test the safety guidelines we had been developing. We beta tested this process at three different hospital programs. This was invaluable because we found that in addition to safety practices, we also needed guidelines that addressed caring for the patient during transport. Our goal in writing these guidelines was to promote teamwork to provide the best patient care in the safest environment.

We found in our peer reviews that medical, aviation, and communications personnel were operating independently and not operating as a team. Medical personnel were practicing patient care based on hospital care guidelines and pilots were following FAA regulations, treating medical teams as passengers instead of as part of a team. Communications was becoming standardized, but as the central point of dispatch and flight following, their importance was often underestimated. Cultural issues were evident. Nurses had always been taught that the patient comes first, completely ignoring their own safety. For example, an important FAA regulation is that all crew and passengers on board must be secured for takeoffs and landings. When we asked nurses what they did if the patient was in cardiac arrest or needed immediate attention during these critical phases of flight, most replied that it was their duty to take care of the patient and they usually undid their seatbelts if they could not reach what they needed.

On the other hand, most of the pilots in those days were pilots with Vietnam experience. These pilots often had as little as 200 hours training before they were sent to Vietnam where completing the mission was their mantra. *(Reference Chapter 3)*

In 1989, I completed the feasibility study to develop an accreditation process based on the principles of the *Joint Commission* on *Accreditation of Healthcare Organizations* (JCAHO), the non-profit agency that accredits hospitals since the 1950s. Part of my study was to engage JCAHO (now known as the Joint Commission) in a presentation to incorporate helicopter air ambulance standards in their accreditation. At the time, most of the helicopter programs were hospital-based. But JCAHO wanted no part of it because they did not have aviation experience or anyone on their Board with an aviation background. I then presented my study to the ASHBEAMS Board and members in October 1989. They voted to provide a loan of $78,000 to a new organization called the Commission on Accreditation of Air Medical Services (CAAMS) to offer accreditation for rotor wing and fixed-wing medical transport services.[6]

This new non-profit organization was set up with a Board of Directors comprised of representatives from the following professional organizations: the National Flight Nurses Association (NFNA), Association of Air Medical Services (AAMS), National Association of Air Communications Specialists (NAACS), American College of Emergency Physicians (ACEP), National EMS Pilots Association (NEMSPA), and the National EMS Physicians Association (NAEMSP). Dr. Nicholas Benson, representing ACEP, became Chair of the Board and I was hired as the Executive Director. We grew from six member organizations to twenty member organizations, representing every discipline involved in medical transport.

In the first several years of developing CAAMS accreditation, there was no income, so we were careful with costs and concentrated on setting up the legal foundation. The internet and social media were certainly not as developed as they are today. Dr. Benson and I tried to get on the speaker's roster at every pertinent EMS or helicopter conference opportunity. In the early years, the aviation operators were not very welcoming of yet another oversight agency. They felt they were already overregulated between the FAA and State licensing. It took many years to convince the aviation professionals that CAAMS was not regulatory, and we were all on the same page – we all wanted to improve safety. As pilots and managers became involved in serving on committees, especially the standards committee, we were able to build trust and respect among all the disciplines involved in air medical transport.

I do not reference fixed wing accidents in this publication. There have been medical transport accidents with airplanes, and we address many of the same issues in standards under the fixed wing section as under the rotor wing section. But airplanes are inherently in a more stable environment because they have controllers and usually file flight plans whereas most helicopters, especially before year 2000, were flying single pilot under Visual Flight Rules (VFR) and not filing flight plans. In fact, there have been many advances in technology over the past 20 years compared to the first years of Helicopter Emergency Medical Services (HEMS) operations.. Today, the FAA uses the term Helicopter Air Ambulance (HAA) instead of HEMS, but you will see it referenced either way.

In 1997, the name changed to Commission on Accreditation of Medical Transport Services (CAMTS). CAAMS always included rotor wing and fixed wing standards, but we started to include ground critical care standards because many pediatric and neonatal teams petitioned our Board of Directors about their safety concerns. These specialty transports are predominantly done by ground ambulance and the hospital usually contracts with an outside agency to provide the ambulance and operator. There were many common ground safety issues: fatigued operators, inappropriate use of red lights and sirens, lack of training etc. that we address in the standards.[8]

The HEMS industry continued a rapid pace of growth, however, that led to more accidents and fatalities. This led to a special investigation by the NTSB in 2006 titled "Special Investigation Report on Emergency Medical Services Operations." Forty-one HEMS accidents and 14 fixed wing EMS accidents were studied that occurred in the previous three years. Few new causes were found. The recurring theme of inclement weather at night and landing in unfamiliar landing sites was evident and only worsened with increased competition and the urgency to respond to patients who are critically ill or injured.

Despite the NTSB's focus on HEMS accidents, 2008 became the deadliest year on record with 8 fatal accidents that resulted in 29 fatalities. The NTSB held a public hearing, and I was called on as an expert witness along with 40 other representatives from FAA Part 135 operators, hospital programs, manufacturers, and associations. Some of the recommendations that resulted were already in the CAMTS accreditation standards. Unlike the lengthy federal government process, a voluntary process such as accreditation has only a Standards Committee, and a board approval process to pass new standards.

The NTSB is required by Congress to investigate every civil accident in all modes of transportation to determine probable causes. However, the NTSB is advisory, not regulatory, so their recommendations to the FAA may or may not be accepted. For example, the NTSB Recommendation A-09-95 to the FAA was to require helicopter emergency medical services operators to install night vision imaging systems, commonly known as night vision goggles or NVGs, and require pilots to be trained in their use during night operations. However, the NTSB recommendation was classified as Closed-Unacceptable Action because the FAA did not include it as a requirement in the February 2014 helicopter rule.

Night Vision Imaging Systems, were strongly encouraged in the 8th Edition. CAMTS Accreditation Standards that were published in 2010 and became a requirement in later editions of the standards. We will be publishing the 12th Edition in 2022.

I have developed a great deal of respect for the NTSB and its Board members who share our mission to improve safety for crews and patients in the air medical environment. We carefully watch the NTSB Most Wanted List and recommendations and share our findings and concerns.

Recent NTSB recommendations on the Most Wanted List include topics such as flight risk tools prior to accepting a flight, comprehensive flight dispatch procedures, use of technologies such as terrain awareness systems (TAWS), Night Vision Imaging Systems (NVIS), Flight Simulator Training, etc. and can be found on the www.ntsb.gov website.

Summary

CAMTS celebrated its 30th Anniversary in 2020. I have had the privilege to meet and know so many caring professionals throughout my nursing career, and especially over the past 30 years.

I want to spotlight three special innovators who had key roles in developing the helicopter air ambulance profession we know today. Please enjoy their personal journeys and contributions to this historical account!

References

1. Collett, H. (1990, July). Mid-year report. *The Journal of Air Medical Transport,* 9(7), i.20.
2. Frazer, E. (2018). *My first flight.* In P. Corbett, A. Wolfe. *A Legacy of Caring: Generations of Critical Care Transport.* Aurora, CO: ASTNA.
3. Frazer, R.S. (1999). Air medical accidents - a 20-year search for information. *AirMed,* 5(5), pp.34-39.
4. Moriarity, R. (1987). Aeromedical safety-a survey – Part 1. *AeroMedical Journal,* 2(5), pp. 50-59.
5. NTSB. (1988). SAFETY STUDY. *Commercial Emergency Medical Service Helicopter Operations.* [NTSB/SS-88/01]. Washington, DC: National Transportation Safety Board.
6. Benson, N., Frazer, E. (1991, November). CAAMS - Developing a voluntary accreditation process. *JEMS,* pp.68-74.
7. Frazer, E. (2020, January/February). Ask the CAMTS AMTC 2019. *Air Medical Journal.* 39(1): 5.
8. Commission on Accreditation of Medical Transport Systems (CAMTS). (2018). *Eleventh Edition Accreditation Standards.* Anderson, SC: CAMTS.

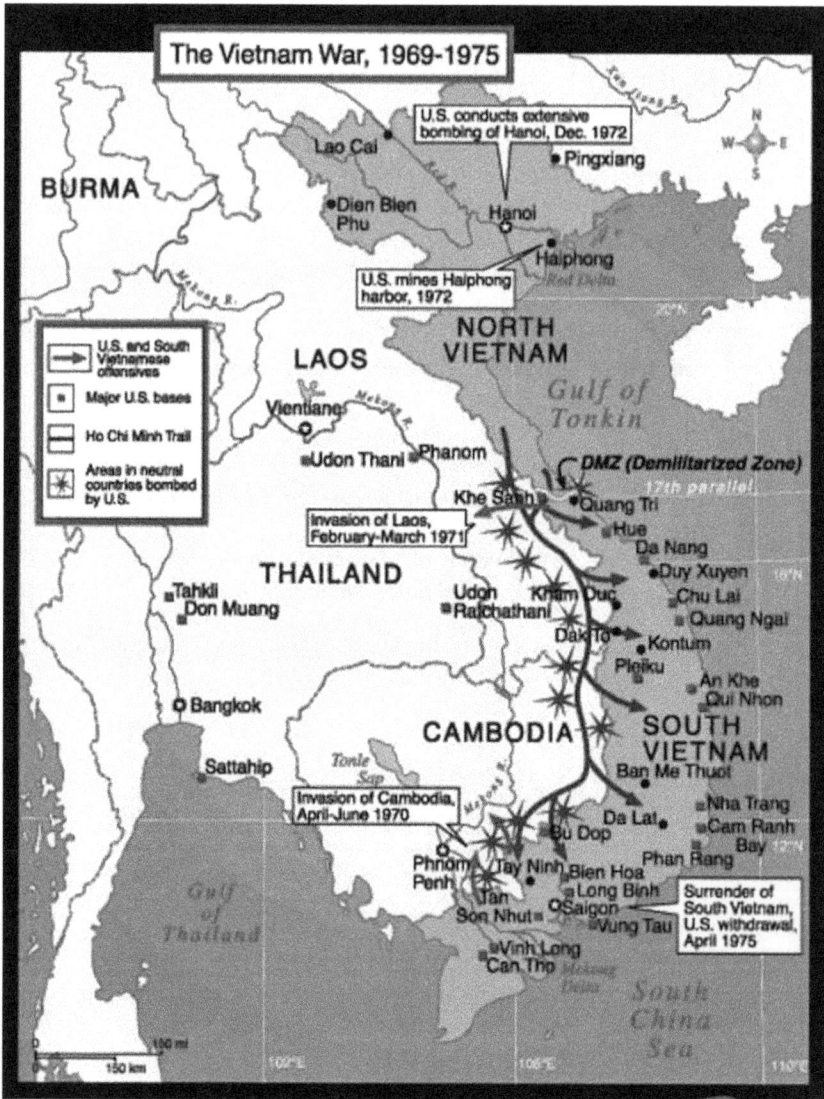

The Geography of the Vietnam War – Lessons – Blendspace

Chapter Two

Marius Burke, the Cuban Missile Crisis and the Vietnam Experience

Marius Burke had several close encounters in American military history, playing a prominent role in the time and space from a top-secret spy mission in Cuba to Air America's part of the Vietnam War. The timing of his military career is an important part of this chapter. Marius started as a Marine Corps pilot in 1958, traveling the world mainly aboard ships. In 1962, he was sent to Guantanamo Bay, Cuba to take over a detachment that flew security using HRS-3 (early Sikorsky S-55) helicopters.

Marius's account of the Cuban Missile Crisis
"I was coming up on my service obligation completion and unfortunately concurrently going through a difficult divorce situation. This put a cloud over me that did not bode well for a long-term career in the Marine Corps. Thus, my plans were to get out as scheduled and go back to school.

Being a "short timer" and readily available, I was asked to go on Temporary Duty to Guantanamo Bay and take over the aviation detachment there. This seemed like a good fit and having been there on several visits during cruises, I looked forward to it and arrived in early August. After a quick checkout in the HRS-3 helicopter given by Bob Ilzhofer, the departing detachment officer, I was clear to go. The unit consisted of two ancient and gutless HRS-3s, four pilots and four maintenance experts. Our mission was to fly around the perimeter of the base, haul VIPs and other visitors around and do whatever else might come up. We had a good tight-knit crew.

As I recall we had no TVs, radios, newspapers, etc. We were, for all practical purposes, out of touch with what was going on in the world. It was quite nice. We did our thing and the only person I communicated with was the airfield boss, Navy Commander Holmgard, who was a good guy and looked out for us Marines.

As previously mentioned, our aircraft were old, and it was a challenge to keep them in the air. Radios were a big problem and they only worked about half of the time. To get around this, if the radios were not working, we would taxi in front of the tower, pull up into a high hover, and give hand signals which the tower folks understood and off we would go. On one of my early flights, I used this procedure, and all worked well until my return when I was notified to immediately report to the Executive/Safety Officer, Lt. Cmdr. Thornley. In any case, I spent the next 15 minutes getting chewed out for not making proper radio contact with the tower. However, in the middle of this process, Cmdr. Holmgard stuck his head in the door and asked me what I was doing. I replied I was in the process of getting chewed out, to which he replied: "Well, when you are done, stop by my house for dinner." I am sure he did it on purpose as he knew what his Executive Officer was like. Also, only he and the Exec. were checked out in a nice Beechcraft T-34 Mentor military trainer aircraft. The earlier versions of the T-34, dating from around the late 1940s to the 1950s, were piston-engine airplanes. He directed Thornley, much to his chagrin, to also check me out. A fun time for me! Not so much for Thornley, though.

After a trip to Guantanamo for R&R, I was informed that my old squadron was sending me a copilot, parachutes and oxygen equipment for a top-secret project using the Sikorsky HR25 (a single radial engine utility helicopter). My only point of contact was to be the Admiral of the base. We worked with a team who introduced themselves as coming from MIT and arrived with $10 million dollars' worth of electronic equipment that filled up the entire cabin. Back in those days, $10 million dollars was worth something. They were not very talkative but said we were to fly up and down the coast of Cuba a mile or so offshore at 10,000 feet. Our first flight was on the 22nd of September. Unfortunately, because of the extremely heavy electronics on board, it was necessary to use much higher power settings just to get off the ground and climb. We were unable to hover and had to make rolling takeoffs due to the weight of the electronics. This would be realized with no warning other than a loud bang and an immediate engine shutting down. Not a good thing! Fortunately, this usually happened when we were at a relatively high altitude, and we were able to slow our descent with the other engine and make it back to Guantanamo.

Upon landing, I called my old squadron and requested they send me a quick engine change. I was told that they had no spare engines. I then called the Admiral and explained our problem. The next morning a C-130 arrived with an engine and we were back in business. That is when I realized the high priority nature of our project. It turned out that the commanding officer of my old squadron was apparently ordered to remove an engine from one of his operating aircraft. In the ensuing days we lost several more engines and went through the same routine. Obviously, this was a high priority project, but we were not told the actual purpose. We went through a few more engine changes over the next few weeks and made it back OK each time.

Given all the maintenance problems we had with the HR2s, and in meeting with the crews, I jokingly called the aircraft a white elephant and said it should be painted white. The next morning, I arrived at the hangar and there was my helicopter with the auxiliary tanks and tail already white! When asked about it later, I simply said it was for identification purposes.

One day we were asked to fly to Navassa Island which is about 100 miles East of Guantanamo and owned by the U.S. A small island only about 1 mile in diameter, it had been occupied in the late 1800s but then abandoned. But they left some goats behind which had multiplied since then. The "MIT" crew set up antennas and did their thing. Unfortunately, shortly after departing we experienced another instantaneous engine failure. Unable to maintain altitude or return to the island, I instructed them to jettison all their equipment which enabled us to just barely make it back to Guantanamo. Obviously, that ended the project. Two weeks later, one of our U-2's was shot down over Cuba. The pilot, Major Rudy Anderson, became the only American killed during the October 1962 Cuban missile crisis. I've often wondered why they (Cuban military) never seemed to have bothered us. They probably couldn't believe we were doing what we were doing.

My completion of active-duty date was 30 October, so I began the checking out process. Two days later, I was called in by my Commanding Officer (C.O.) to inform me that due to the Cuban Missile crisis, everyone had been put on indefinite duty extension. I proceeded to check back in but then there was a clarification saying anyone scheduled to get out prior to 31 October would get out as scheduled. I was due to get out on 30 October. Once again I met with my C.O. and after much discussion I told him if I could be assigned to the new Iwo Jima helicopter carrier (which was air conditioned) and go in on the first wave, I would extend. Foolish me! In any

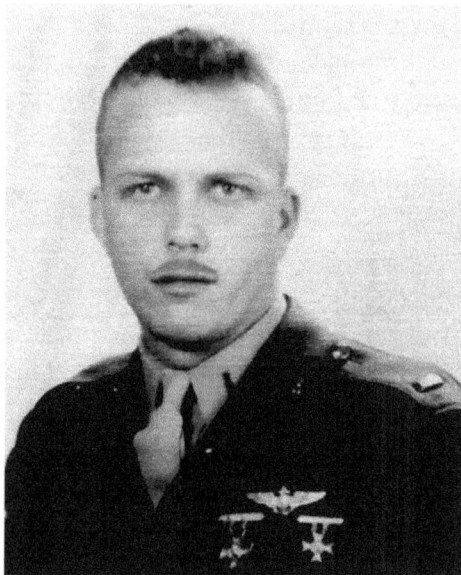

Marius in full military uniform in early 1960s

case, we ended up milling around the Caribbean for a few months with no action and finally returned home. Of course, I was now on an indefinite extension which no one seemed to know what to do about, but finally I was asked to give them a date. I did and got out on 30 January 1963.

My plan was to finish up my degree and since I had established residence in North Carolina, I signed up at East Carolina College. Residence tuition was very reasonable, and it looked like things were working out as school was going well. However, towards the end of the first quarter, I was called in by the Dean who was also a Marine, but not an aviator. He proceeded to tell me that although I met all the requirements for residency, he did not think I would be staying in North Carolina after I finished. All my arguments fell on deaf ears, so after that quarter I had to leave. I then signed up at North Carolina State as a resident. But I was flagged again at the end of the quarter and told that since East Carolina had declared me to be a non-resident, they had no choice but to do the same.

Under those conditions, I was left with no choice but to find a job and make enough money to go back to school. Less than a week later I received a call from a fellow in Washington, D.C. offering me a flying job overseas. Apparently, the "MIT" folks must have flagged me as a person who might be talked into doing stupid and dangerous things and they somehow tracked me. Thus, my next great adventure was to begin with Air America."

Air America and more aviation adventures in Southeast Asia

The well-kept secret about Air America was that it was owned by the CIA since the late 1940s. According to Allen Cates, author of *Honor Denied*,[1] the history of the war in Southeast Asia would not be complete if Air America is excluded. Air America was certainly visible and known to the locals but as news of Vietnam appeared in ever increasing intensity in the late 1960s, there was little known about Air America–an entity that resided in this part of the world for at least twenty-five years. If portrayed at all, as in the movie production starring Mel Gibson, Air America pilots and crews were mercenaries, profiteers, and crazy daredevils. The government did not discourage or contradict this unfair reputation because Air America was a secret support arm of the CIA, and the military and government did not want this disclosed to the public.

Most of the Air America staff was not there to be rich and famous or infamous. The secretive nature of this organization prevented airmen and support crews from collecting military aid, healthcare, and pensions because they fell into an abyss of neither military nor civil service.[2] Cate's book tells of the struggles to achieve the same benefits and recognition as the military who were fighting the same war from the same country – whether under a cloak of secrecy or in the open on the nightly news. These individuals all suffered and died at the same time and space. The Director of National Intelligence's report in 2011 rejected federal benefits because Air America workers never thought they were government employees. For those surviving Air America veterans who are U.S. citizens, an estimated 380 according to a 2017 story in the *Star Tribune*,[2] this struggle for equal benefits continues. A Senate bill, sponsored by 13 senators last year failed to change this policy. However, there are still counsels for Air America working to earn civil service benefits for these survivors.

When Marius joined Air America, they flew Sikorsky H 34 helicopters and his status was 1st Officer, then promoted to Captain. Marius also flew airplanes. His Southeast Asia experiences at this tumultuous time with a secretive military arm of the CIA can best be described by his own narrative as follows.

Marius Burke - In his own words:

"Initially, I was based in Udorn, Thailand, while the overall Chief Pilot was in Taipei. Since Air America was recognized as an airline, we had customers. These were people paying for travel and some were CIA agents. Many of these agents were great folks but some were just flat-out crazy.

Air America flew many missions behind enemy lines. These dangerous missions were up to the pilot and leadership did not mind if the odds were against them – pilots were expendable. One of the more colorful customers was the legendary Anthony Poshepny, more commonly referred to as Tony Po. It seems that he was loosely portrayed in the role of Col. Walter Kurtz in the movie "Apocalypse Now" and played by Marlon Brando. Tony had a vast amount of experience dating back to Korea and was a real tough but straight-shooting individual. I enjoyed working with him and never felt he put me in unnecessary harms' way. If there was any doubt in his mind about a mission, he would either tell me I was not going or that he was going with me. He never let me down.

We normally flew single-pilot and were always challenged by the weather and terrain. There were three seasons: Smokey, Rainy and Clear. We had an Automatic Direction Finder (ADF) but there were no Global Positioning Systems (GPSs) etc. at that time and little other navigation aids – so we were mostly flying by time and heading. There were no power lines to worry about. But, in addition to the challenging mountainous terrain and changing weather conditions, there were guns on the ground and always the possibility of being shot down.

Pilots were required to call in every 30 minutes (we had VHF and HF radios) and if they did not hear from you in 60 minutes, they would start looking for you. At one point, I was trapped in a line of thunderstorms returning to base one evening. The only route open was over the Plain Des Jayres, which was held by the enemy and full of anti-aircraft weapons. I wound up climbing to 20,000 feet and got above the clouds. Of course, there was no oxygen equipment, and the regulation states oxygen is needed if flying 30 minutes or more above 10,000 feet. But after about 15 minutes, I was able to let down and made it back to our upcountry main base to fly another day.

My initial flight pay as a First officer was $650.00 per month plus a small hourly flight stipend. After a few months, when I was upgraded to Captain, it was raised to $1,050 per month. Adequate housing was $500.00 a month minimally. At first, most of us resided with one or two other pilots to share expenses. American food was very expensive and on that salary one could not afford a car. Cars were taxed at 300%, so most of us used bicycles or motorcycles to get around. The company provided transportation to and from the base. While the types of missions we flew certainly commanded risk taking, it was something most of us looked forward to. Sadly, given the low pay and expenses, many of my peers left with little or no more than what they possessed when they arrived.[3]

When we signed on for Air America, full physicals and immunizations for yellow fever and tuberculosis were required. There was a clinic on the base staffed by one nurse. We had two Chinese physicians who were also FAA examiners at Headquarters in Taipei, and they would come twice a year to give physicals to the pilots. We had a long list of immunizations, and we were prescribed quinine tablets daily for malaria. Unfortunately, one of our flight mechanics went home on leave and died two weeks later of a ruptured spleen, supposedly caused by malaria. The quinine had apparently masked the symptoms. I stopped taking the tablets after that, thinking that if I contracted malaria I wanted to know about it. If we needed more extensive medical care, we would go to the Bangkok Christian Hospital in Bangkok. A number of our folks contracted hepatitis resulting in a stay at this hospital. I had been working out of the Bangkok office and not upcountry and I was one of the fortunate few. The only significant medical problem I had was a bout with dengue fever which knocked me out for a few weeks.

Air America operated many aircraft makes and models from a Bell 47 to a Convair 880. At the time, I believe United Airlines was the only airline that had more aircraft than Air America. Before I arrived, Air America was also operating some Sikorsky H-19s, but they were unsuited for mountainous terrain. Amazingly, the company decided to check out senior pilots who were not helicopter qualified in these aircraft but that did not go well. They all crashed. In 1961, the Marine Corps sent a detachment to Udorn flying Sikorsky H-34s. They did some flying in Laos. But after about 6 months, they were given the option to stay in the Marine Corps or work for Air America. Three or four of the pilots decided to work for Air America and the H-34s were given to the company. So, these were military aircraft, and we received more H-34s as needs increased.

Many aircraft in Air America's fleet were Chinese registered such as C-47, C-46. Other aircraft, including a Bell 47, were not Chinese registered. It was no easy task to get these aircraft Chinese registered because the Taiwanese did not want to give us licenses. Air America was a commercial operation, flying scheduled flights throughout the Far East. We were also the flag carrier for Taiwan, which was granted during the days of Clair Chenault. But Taiwan now had its own airline that was not a flag carrier for Taiwan.

Air America eventually received new Bell UH1H helicopters that were slated for the military. These aircraft were up to military standards but not FAA standards. They were designated Bell 205s and we ended up getting them Laos registered. This required Laos licenses that were much easier to get compared to Chinese licenses. The last Chinese license I got was a 3–4-day ordeal.

In juggling these aircraft and licenses, it was discovered that one of the former Marine pilots never had a U.S. pilot's license. He had to go back to the U.S. to get a license, after flying several years with no license at all.

In 1974, we shut down operations in Laos. I arrived in Saigon in June 1974 and was sent to Da Nang in early March 1975 to take over the base operations there. I had worked there on a few previous occasions and looked forward to the change of venue.

The Da Nang Air America base normally housed four helicopters and one or two fixed wing aircraft. There were three Bell 204Bs and one Bell UH1H which was dedicated to the International Control Commission Services (ICCS). The ICCS was composed of representatives from Poland and Hungary who essentially represented the North Vietnamese interests and the Indonesians and Iranians who represented the South Vietnamese/U.S. interests. Their mission was supposedly to monitor the "cease fire" or "peace accords." This often required transporting them behind enemy lines. Air America had this contract. The dedicated aircraft were painted with ICCS logos, etc., for recognition purposes. When pilots worked this contract, they wore different insignia and hats. Pilots and crews were interchangeable between carrying ICCS personnel and our "regular" missions. A year or so earlier, on an ICCS trip behind enemy lines, the two assigned helicopters were shot down. Everyone was killed on one, but the other aircraft managed to land safely. All personnel were taken prisoner and held for a few days before being released.

Initially, operations at Da Nang were relatively benign. However, on the 17th of March 1975 things started to change. Reports began coming in regarding heavier than normal unfriendly activity between Hue and Quang Tri to the north. The more information that was received, the less inclined I was to launch the scheduled ICCS helicopter to Quang Tri that morning. Contact was made with the Indonesian Air Operations representative of the ICCS to discuss the matter. He blandly informed me that a chopper was not required. Apparently the military situation had gotten so bad that all the ICCS delegates had abandoned Quang Tri the night before and had gone by road to Hue but failed to inform Air America of the situation. It is fortunate I contacted the Indonesians before we sent the scheduled helicopter to an area that had likely been overrun!

Reports continued to come in regarding activity north of Hue, which indicated the possible presence of North Vietnamese tanks in the area but there seemed to be little other apparent concern. Some pressure was expected to be put on Hue, but the word put out by the "customer" was that it was nothing to be alarmed about. On the 18th of March, the first enemy shelling was experienced at Hue. I recommended to the OSA customer that their representatives in Hue should be brought back to Da Nang each evening. They disagreed. Thus, the tone for future events was set.

At about 7PM on the 19th, a call was received from Roy Lewis (OSA Operations Manager) stating that there was an emergency at Hue due to heavy shelling and reported nearby tank activity. He wanted helicopters sent up to evacuate his people. Since normal flying activities were limited to daytime operations, this was truly considered an emergency. Two crews were organized and departed about 8PM. Upon arrival at Hue, they had to wait for some time since not everyone was ready to go. Finally, the last stragglers showed up and they headed back to Da Nang. Some ground fire was received on the return trip, but it could not be determined if it was friendly or unfriendly.

Upon returning to Da Nang, a request was received from the ICCS delegation to evacuate their personnel from Hue. They again launched, arriving at Hue around 9:30 PM and waited for almost 45 minutes for passengers to show up. None did. By this point they were at a low fuel state and had to depart. They were told the next day that these personnel had not finished packing and that was why they did not show up! Obviously, their sense of urgency was far less than Air America crew members.

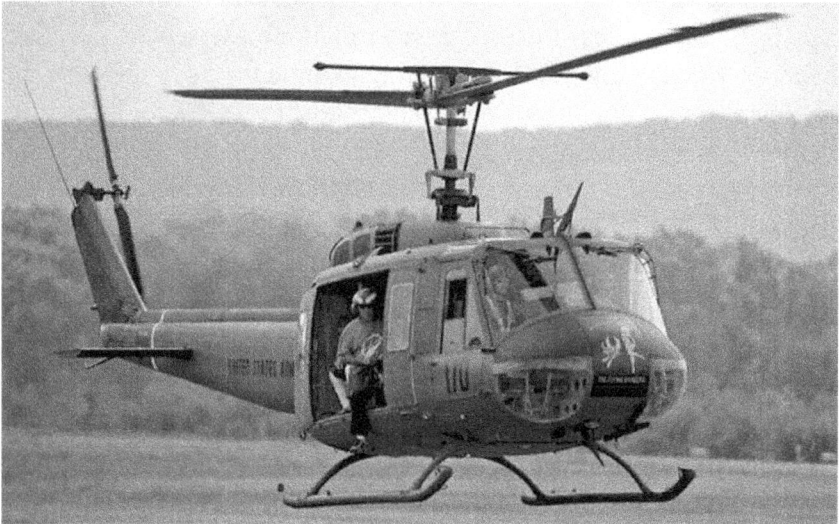

Bell UH-1H (Huey) widely used in Viet Nam (courtesy Times Leader)

On 20 March, the situation at Hue appeared to be less tenuous. Customers were going to Hue in the morning and returning to Da Nang in the evening. However, it was noted that refugees were filtering South in ever increasing numbers. This exodus increased as shelling of Hue began once more. Finally, on the 23rd of March, an urgent call was received to evacuate all remaining customers due to heavy enemy activity. This was accomplished.

The weather had been very marginal during those past few days; ceilings were running from 20 to 100 feet with rain throughout the area. One helicopter was launched for Quang Ngai (about a 30-minute flight south of Da Nang) early in the morning with customers for what was considered normal administrative purposes. As they approached Quang Ngai they were told by people on the ground that they were taking fairly heavy mortar fire and it was recommended they not land. The customers on board assured the pilots that even with the incoming mortars they still wanted to be put on the ground and this was accomplished. They then headed for the coast and north to drop other customers off at Tam Ky. At this point they encountered very heavy rain and discovered their windshield wipers were inoperative. Since the drop off at Tam Ky was not considered urgent, they decided to head back to Da Nang for repairs. Minutes later, a panic call was received from the customers at Quang Ngai that they now wanted to be pulled out as soon as possible.

I was getting ready to take a mission to Hue when they received notice that Tam Ky had fallen to the enemy overnight and almost simultaneously received a call from Izzy regarding his maintenance problems and the evacuation requirements at Quang Ngai. I then launched for Quang Ngai to pick up the customers there. Another pilot headed to Hue on that mission. He had two demolition experts whose job was to bring down the Voice of America Towers located several miles south of the Citadel. This was to prevent the enemy from using the station for propaganda if Hue were lost. They were supposed to be joined by two Vietnamese Chinook helicopters that were carrying troops to secure the area while the demolition folks did their thing. The Vietnamese helicopters never showed up. While awaiting clearance from the customer to drop their passengers off at the towers, they went and landed at the Province Pad located just across the river from the Citadel.

To their surprise, they found people still manning the site. They were mostly Filipino communications personnel. Since everyone else had been evacuated, it seemed prudent to pull them out. They were taken to an airstrip just south of the Perfume River on the beach. While enroute, the customer called and advised them that under no circumstances should anyone be put on the ground at the VOA site without Vietnamese troops there for security. By this time, I had

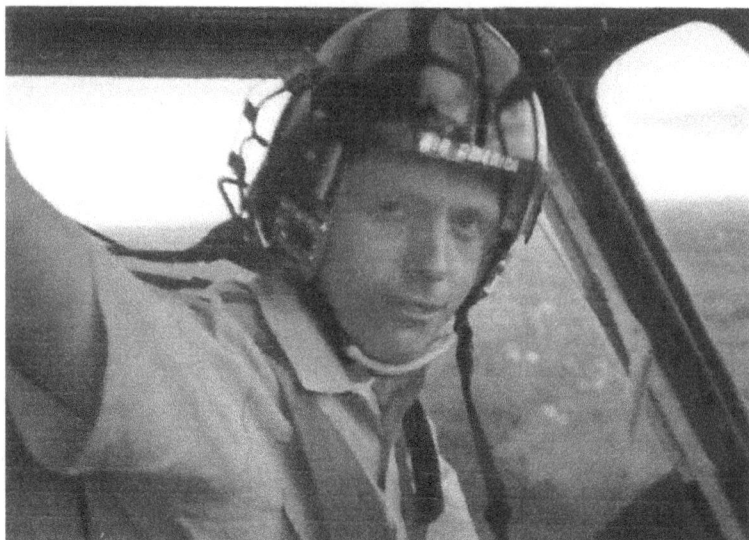

Marius flying in Vietnam - year not identified

pulled the folks out of Quang Ngai and proceeded to Hue where we evacuated the rest of the people needing to come out. Interestingly, Hue appeared to be in control, with armor and artillery heading from Camp Edwards to the Citadel to make a stand. However, in the morning we sent a Volpar up to see how things looked and they saw the North Vietnamese flag flying over the Citadel. A few days later, the North Vietnamese were broadcasting from the VOA with a different message - so much for planning and communications.

On the 25th, shortly after receiving the news from the Volpar flight, a call was received from the Polish representative of the ICCS wanting us to schedule a flight to Hue that afternoon. The Indonesians were responsible for scheduling all aviation operations for the ICCS, so I reminded him that was the protocol. Additionally, he was told that Hue was now under the control of the enemy. His reaction was confusing until I realized that I was essentially speaking with the enemy! After some additional discussion he informed me that I didn't understand his request and that they were willing to pay us to fly them in our company aircraft. When he started talking about how much they were willing to pay, I told him this was not a negotiating point. Nevertheless, he indicated that a call would be made later with a better offer. That did not happen.

That same day, a recon flight was made with the objective of finding alternate safe landing destinations in the event an evacuation of Da Nang became necessary. The closest satisfactory safe area appeared to be the islands approximately ten miles off the coast of Da Nang which were occasionally used as bombing ranges. However, the U.S. Consul General in Da Nang, Al Francis, felt that security at the islands was questionable even at that time and my plans to position fuel there were quashed.

It soon became obvious that our non-essential personnel needed to be evacuated from Da Nang. Although extra company aircraft were coming up to take people out, there generally were no extra seats for our employees. A seat belt waiver was requested to allow more people on board each aircraft, but it was not authorized. It took what seemed forever to convey the seriousness of the situation to the folks in Saigon. Finally, a waiver was granted, and we were able to legally (at least by the company) add more people to the departing flights.

Nevertheless, we still encountered difficulties getting company personnel and dependents on the airlifts. In fact, at one time I was told by a U.S. Consulate official that Air America personnel had no right to ride on departing Air America aircraft but rather should go by boat! With that comment, a short discussion ensued during which I threatened to shut down all Air America operations. Our people were finally given appropriate consideration.

Just before dawn on the 26th, about 400 refugees from Quang Tri and Hue appeared on our ramp and informed me that they were waiting to go out on the airlift heading south, which was now in full swing. They stated that they were given approval to come aboard the air base by the Base Security Officer. I managed to convince them to clear the ramp and they then set up camp outside our gate. As the airlift progressed, this crowd seemed to act as a catalyst and soon the numbers grew to thousands. They then began breaking through the barriers we had erected to keep the ramp clear for arriving aircraft. Two Vietnamese generals on the scene were asked to control the crowd but their only reply was that they were incapable of doing anything about the situation. I'm sure the only reason they were there was to make sure their families got out on the airlift. Seeing these two Generals just standing around while their country was being invaded, cemented my feelings that the end was near.

Communications and coordination between my office and the customer warehouse next door became increasingly difficult and reached the point where I was forced to literally take over all air operations functions. There was a ten-foot wall separating our buildings, but our offices were literally less than ten feet apart. Games had to be played because the ramp was now overrun with refugees. Arriving and departing aircraft were told to park at various areas on the field, then passengers were bussed out to the aircraft. Finally, the Consul General, Al Francis, attempted to appease the refugees by dedicating the next arriving 727 solely for their use if they would promise to maintain order. This gambit failed, with the result that on the 27th he called off the World Airways airlift. Attempts were still made by our company aircraft, with marginal success. By this time, the VNAF (Vietnamese Air Force) had compromised all our radio frequencies and as soon as an aircraft landed, they would be hot on its heels with a caravan of vehicles loaded with their people to scramble to the aircraft.

In the past, I had requested that our N registered X-Ray Bell 204B's (8 passenger capacity and small fuel tanks with resulting short range) be replaced by the Foxtrot H modes which had greater passenger and fuel capacity and thus longer-range capabilities. Only one of the three was replaced. In the end, we had one ICCS H model and two X-Ray Bell 204Bs.

This created problems as we now needed to rescue more people and fly greater distances in this risky environment. In addition, I was given specific instructions from Saigon that we were not to utilize the ICCS H model Bell for anything but official ICCS missions.

It was decided to cut operations personnel to the absolute minimum and keep only one pilot per aircraft and no flight attendants or flight mechanics, planning instead to utilize the Filipino ground mechanics who could do double duty and who also had good local contacts. However, it appeared that Saigon just didn't realize the seriousness of our situation despite repeated requests that replacement crews and cargo not be sent to Da Nang. There was no longer time to worry about complying with regulations. The crews present were asked to decide whether or not they wished to stay

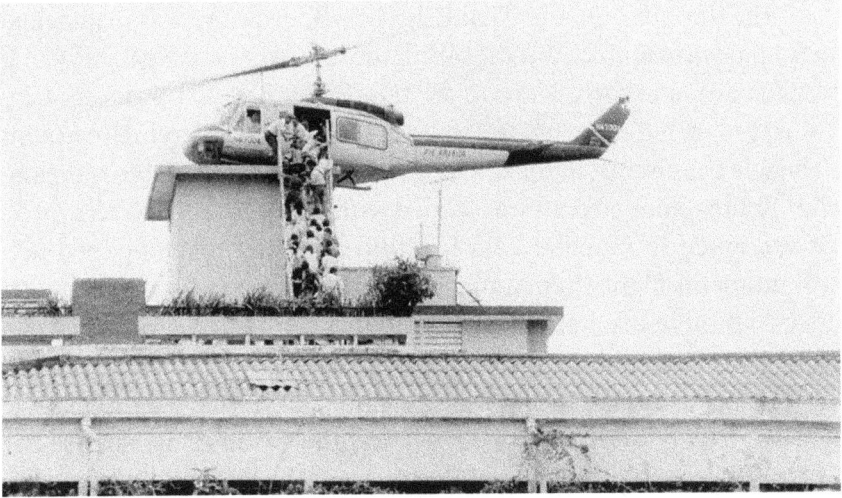

Evacuation of Saigon, Vietnam, April 1975
(Photo Credit Getty Images)

since I planned no reliefs after crews were designated. Terry Olson specifically requested to stay till the end, and the other crews said they would stay if needed. Nevertheless, replacements and cargo continued to show up. Crews were simply loaded back aboard the aircraft and sent home. Unfortunately, this took up seats we could have used for other people having to leave. One night, we worked until midnight unloading unneeded cargo so we could get passengers out first thing in the morning. All of this simply slowed down the airlift and clogged up our ramp.

Fuel was another vital consideration. I fully expected that should the situation deteriorate, Shell Oil would not be available to provide fuel, and we likely could not expect any support from the military (this turned out to be so). A search was made for drummed fuel that we could cache away. None was readily available in Da Nang. Saigon seemed to have little interest in helping us out in this respect, instead referring us back to Shell Oil in Da Nang. After many requests, we finally received 12 empty drums from Saigon that were in such poor condition that only two were usable! We spent many nights searching for empty drums in the area and attempting to salvage them for our purposes. Some of the few we did manage to obtain were eventually put to good use. I was beginning to wonder if Saigon hadn't already been taken over by the other side!

The day after Quang Ngai fell, Mike Braithwaite was dispatched to Saigon with our fifth aircraft. With the loss of Quang Ngai, refueling became a major consideration for the X-Ray Bell 204 models. Chu Lai was reported to be secure, so it was scheduled as a refueling point to enable the aircraft to make Quin Nhon, the next available refueling site. Braithwaite's aircraft was loaded with evacuees and launched. As he attempted to refuel at Chu Lai, unfriendly elements opened fire, wounding his flight attendant and one passenger. He managed to get airborne and return to Da Nang. Among other hits, one was taken in a rotor blade spar and another in the engine, requiring changes of both. By now it was apparent that the situation had reached a critical stage and the ARVN (Vietnamese Army) and the VNAF (Vietnamese Air Force) were doing little or nothing to stem the unfriendly advances. Da Nang was becoming increasingly isolated.

We had one rotor blade in stock but required an engine from Saigon. A request was immediately sent out but despite the arrival of several aircraft that day (incidentally, all loaded with unneeded cargo), no engine showed up. Finally, late the following evening the replacement engine arrived. Much of that night was spent installing and running FCF's (Functional Check Flights). It was again dispatched to Saigon the following day, this time carrying some of the drum fuel we had stashed away so it could bypass Chu Lai.

Despite the tremendous loss of territory surrounding Da Nang, the word from the powers that be was that there would definitely be a stand and the city would not be allowed to fall into enemy hands.

On the night of the 26th, several late evening administrative flights were flown, the last aircraft landing after 8PM. Shell Oil had agreed to retain enough people to support us if we promised to evacuate them when the time came. However, on this evening we ran into problems. Access to our ramp by normal means was blocked off. The only way to get to it was by going to the end of the field and then up the taxiway. The tower refused Shell permission to do this. After much running around, I decided to take the truck myself and drive it through, thinking the VNAF might be more willing to deal with an American. Unfortunately, in the meantime, the Shell driver left with the truck, driving it to their compound and locking it up. This left us with three aircraft in a low fuel state. Not a very desirable situation under the circumstances. After some significant negotiations with the VNAF, permission was given allowing us to refuel across the field at their refueling pits. At this, we breathed a little easier.

On the 27th, the situation was relatively unchanged except that we had literally thousands of people camped out in our operating area. They weren't overly unruly but made it clear they would not leave until an aircraft took them away. Hundreds of people were also camping out in the OSA customer compound and travel between the two areas was almost impossible. That afternoon, after making some local administrative flights, one of the OSA customers got out of my aircraft and left his special radio behind. I decided to hold onto it.

All crews had now been instructed to spend the night at the field. Around 9:00 PM, I attempted to go downtown and retrieve personal belongings as well as those of Frank Stergar. Upon arrival at the gate, I met some of the Filipino mechanics who had been spending the last few nights at the field and had gone downtown to get some of their belongings. The gate was closed except for military traffic and the guards would not let them or their vehicles back on the base. I then walked out of the gate and attempted to drive one of their vehicles in. This resulted in some heated discussions with the gate guards for almost an hour, finally terminating with the guards shooting into the air with their weapons, indicating that discussions were ended. I got the picture. With that, I parked the vehicle and attempted to walk back in. Permission was refused. After another 30 minutes of discussions, they finally let me in but refused the Filipinos entry. I instructed them to go to the company hostel downtown and spend the night. A VHF radio had been installed there for such a situation and they were to check in upon their safe arrival (the phone was no longer working). This was accomplished and they were advised to return to the base in the morning. If that were not possible, we made plans to pick them up at a prearranged spot by helicopter.

Around midnight, a call was received from the hostel stating there was shooting in the neighborhood and houses were being ransacked. The hostel was reputed to be the next target. Instructions were given for all personnel to leave and proceed down the block to the customer OSA motor pool, which was considered secure. I attempted to contact Saigon with these latest developments, but no contact could be made.

For the last week I had been camping out in our administrative office. When I first came up to Da Nang, things were rather busy, and I never bothered getting the safe combination from our Vietnamese accountant. Just the day before, Saigon had delivered that month's payroll and it was sitting in the safe just opposite my cot. The accountant was off base and after the events of the evening, I wished I had gotten the combination should the accountant not be able to return to the base. No telling what else might have been in the safe but certainly things one wouldn't want to leave behind.

At approximately 2:00 AM, the radio that I had "acquired" suddenly came alive. A voice, apparently that of the OSA Chief, Robert Grealy, made a call instructing someone to get his people down to the docks immediately. A few more calls followed and finally the folks in the OSA warehouse next door were asked how many Americans they had at the base. The reply was "13" (it was obvious this did not include us!). They were told to get in a vehicle, leave the base and go to the docks. I waited a short while for the expected call but when it became obvious that none would be forthcoming, I called next door and asked what was going on. The answer was, "I don't know, except we have been told to get off the base." I then asked what we were supposed to do. The reply was, "Do the best you can." When asked if that meant we were on our own, I received an answer in the affirmative. It was at this time that I sent a message to Saigon stating it appeared the end was imminent. The only response I recall was that I was not to use the ICCS helicopter for anything other than ICCS work.

A short while later the OSA group returned saying the gates were closed and they would try in the morning when curfew was lifted at 6AM but that help might be needed from us! It was at this point that I roused the rest of our crews and other employees at the field, informing them preparations were being made to depart. That is, if the many people camped out on the ramp would let us.

The previous day the airstrip at Marble Mountain had been cleared of debris for possible contingency use and time distance planning had been accomplished for what appeared the only viable alternative destination after leaving Da Nang: Cu Le Re Island. This small volcanic looking island about 10 miles off the coast of Chu Lai, was only about a mile in diameter but was renowned for its garlic. It also had a small airstrip.

During the night all our people surreptitiously carried minimal personal belongings out to the helicopters. They then waited behind the hangar. It was planned to attempt departure just prior to first light when most folks would still be half asleep. All four aircraft would start up simultaneously and as soon as that happened, our passengers would then make a run for it, and we would depart... hopefully.

Fortunately, we had enough edge to accomplish just that, although by the time we were lifting off, a huge crowd was heading for us and quite a few were trying to grab the skids as we departed. Fog was just beginning to form. A C-46, almost over Da Nang, was advised of the situation, and asked to attempt a landing at Marble Mountain to pick up our passengers. It landed just prior to the runway being masked completely by fog.

Two more trips were made to the Air America ramp in an attempt to police up any recognizable stragglers. This was difficult in as much as it was necessary to hover over what was now a panicky crowd and try to snatch up only those people we wanted. On the last try, there appeared to be no one else except one of our utility men who kept running away whenever we hovered near him. The rotor washes apparently frightened him more than the fear of being left behind. About this time, some people in the crowd began firing at us and we were forced to depart.

While we were hovering over the crowd looking for employees, mechanic Gil decided to tell me what was sitting inside our locked hangar. Apparently the previous night the paymaster for the German Hospital came to our facility in one of their ambulances. He was a friend of the mechanics. He had the hospital payroll, which was more than $250,000 with him in the ambulance. Apparently, due to all the commotion, he was unable to properly distribute the money. At the same time, he was concerned about having that money with him for fear he would be held up. Thus, the ambulance and the money were locked up in our hangar for safekeeping. I told Gil that under the circumstances, he was welcome to go get it. I would let him off and come back for him. He wisely demurred. It was funny how little money meant at a time like that.

While enroute to Marble Mountain with our load of evacuees, a call was received from our OSA "friends" requesting help since they could not get off the airfield. We were informed that they were being followed by several vehicles full of people whom they could not get away from. Instructions were given for them to reverse course and head for the tennis court area where we would rendezvous and attempt to pick them up before those following could catch up. This was accomplished and their pursuers were discouraged from getting aboard by a display of fire power on the part of our passengers. Everyone was deposited at Marble Mountain where the C-46 was still standing by. All was quiet at this strip and the C-46 departed after being fully loaded. It was reported some days later that the "unfriendly pursuers" were probably indigenous OSA employees. What was most regrettable was that we could have gotten all of them out.

One by one, as we burned down to minimum fuel for the trip to Cu Le Re Island, the helicopters departed. Weather was marginal, with 100–200-foot ceilings and ¼ mile visibility as we proceeded south. I followed the two X-Ray models since my ICCS H model had greater fuel capacity. Vic Carpenter, in 12 Foxtrot, was the last to depart, being 10 minutes behind me. For some reason, he did not feel he could make it to the island because of the weather and returned to Marble Mountain where the weather was a little better. He contacted a Volpar that was overhead and was able to land and pick him up.

The trip to the island was tedious at best. With no navigational facilities, one had to fly strictly time, distance and heading, hoping the island would appear before we ran out of fuel. Fortunately, things worked out and shortly after arrival, the weather cleared up and the Volpar was able to land and join us. It had enough fuel on board to enable us to top off one X-Ray model. Terry Olson volunteered to accompany me back to Da Nang in an attempt to find other personnel. We estimated about 10-15 minutes on station with our fuel load.

Upon arriving in the area, we called the VNAF and asked if they would give us some fuel. Their reply was "No fuel for Americans." We persisted, telling them we were there to help Vietnamese, and after much deliberation, they consented. "But only you and no one else."

We topped off and attempted to recover the helicopter at Marble Mountain. It was still intact, however, in the pilot's haste to leave, he had failed to turn off the battery and it was now dead. Batteries were switched and aircraft started and subsequently refueled. In return for fuel the VNAF required one aircraft to work for them hauling personnel and their dependents from the airfield to Deep Water Pier where barges were docked for evacuation purposes.

During this time contact was made with the Consul General, Al Francis, and I carried him to various places while he attempted to assist in evacuating additional people. While he was visiting the various command posts, we searched the area and located about 30 additional Air America employees and their dependents that had been trapped off base. They were deposited at the boat docks for further evacuation. As it began getting dark, the base fuel pits closed down (apparently out of fuel), and we had to depart.

All attempts to get Mr. Francis to leave with us were fruitless since he had just received information that General Truong, who had the reputation as one of the toughest commanders in Vietnam and one of the most arrogant, was purportedly planning to commit suicide. Francis felt it was his duty to prevent this from happening (I would have let him). We were asked to come back in the morning to pick him up if he hadn't departed by boat at that time. We reluctantly departed for the island where we refueled and proceeded to Nha Trang for the night. Additional drummed fuel had been brought out to the island for our use.

Two Bell helicopters from Nha Trang were loaded with four 55-gallon drums of fuel each for an early morning departure the next day. Ron Goodwin accompanied me with Terry Olson and Tony Coalson flying the other aircraft. There was to be a Volpar C-45 overhead to provide support and communications and a Caribou C-7 was to position additional fuel at the island.

Da Nang was a shambles when we arrived. Aircraft, tanks, trucks, etc., were abandoned all over the area. The aircraft apparently were out of fuel. It appeared that many of the trucks and tanks had been driven into the ocean in an attempt to connect with boats and ships offshore. Rockets were impacting the airfield and small arms fire was received from all areas of the city. The Consulate was on fire. A search was commenced for Mr. Francis with no success. Finally, a large group of people was spotted in the French compound. A note was dropped to them asking the whereabouts of Francis and telling them to proceed to Landing Zone 48, which was the nearest landing area if they wanted to be picked up. Shortly thereafter, some vehicles departed the compound and headed for LZ 48. Upon arriving, they were turned back due to large crowds and small arms fire. They returned to the compound.

Since there was no room to land, Olson and Coalson made a low pass, snatching two Frenchmen on the skids. Quite a bit of fire was received from the area surrounding the compound as well as from the tanks that were outside the walls. The two evacuees had some interesting stories to relate regarding the previous night's happenings but had no knowledge of Francis' whereabouts. They were not overly concerned about the fate of their compatriots who were left behind, saying, "We Frenchmen can get along with these people."

We eventually landed on a small sandbar in the middle of Da Nang harbor to hot refuel from the drum fuel on board using hand pumps. VNAF personnel were constantly calling upon us with their survival radios to pick them up. We were continuing our search over the city when suddenly a 727 was spotted turning base for landing. All frequencies, including Guard, were tried in an attempt to make contact and warn them not to land. No response was received. The aircraft landed and stopped about three quarters of the way down the runway. It was immediately surrounded by troops and vehicles (at this time only a few civilians could be seen at the airfield but there were thousands of military troops). About five minutes later the pilots began communicating with the tower. Only at that time did the crew finally acknowledge our transmissions. They had apparently been reading us all along but chose not to answer.

This was a World Airways aircraft with their President, Ed Daly, on board. They had apparently been refused permission to take off from Saigon but did so anyway. In what appeared to be a grandstand play, they had their Traffic Manager and a UP photographer on board who was supposed to record this "lifesaving" mission. When asked what they were doing, the crew responded, "You wouldn't believe us if we told you." My reply was that they better take off and get out right away if they could. No response. They then taxied to the south end of runway 17 Left and were again surrounded. By now the runway was littered with bodies and overturned vehicles. I suggested they go to runway 35 Left and take off as it was relatively open, although there was still some sporadic incoming in the area. A noncommittal response was again given. About this time, I really didn't think they had a chance of getting off the ground and was trying to figure out how we could possibly pull them out by helicopter. It looked hopeless.

Suddenly, a panicked American voice came up on the radio from the tower. He identified himself as Joe Hrezo and screamed for someone to save him. More problems! Apparently, he and the UP photographer had deplaned to assist with loading and recording the event. Unfortunately, they were unable to get back on board due to the mob trying to get on board. With this the 727 taxied down the runway, across to the taxiway in front of the tower and stopped at midfield.

About 20-30 seconds passed at which time I informed them that both runways were now unusable, and their only chance was to take off on the taxiway they were on. "We think you're right," was heard from the 727 and with that they began a takeoff roll. As it started rolling, they narrowly missed a stalled van on the side of the taxiway but a motorcycle coming from the opposite direction smashed into the aircraft, hurling its driver into the infield. The aircraft was still on the ground as it ran off the end of the taxiway but somehow became airborne after blowing through several small structures at the end of the field.

It was some time after they took off before we could get a report if Hrezo had made it on board or not. Finally, they called saying he was on board. However, it seemed the UP photographer had been left behind and we were asked to pick him up. But where…and how? Small arms fire was again picking up as we let down in an effort to spot this individual. Finally, the photographer made it to the tower and began calling for help. He was instructed to go to the far end of the field, which was relatively deserted at the time. We would try to make a pickup there. He departed and the Vietnamese tower operator kept us apprised of his progress until he was out of his sight. The tower operator pleaded with us to save the photographer, saying we were his only chance of getting out.

We made a low-level run to see if we could spot our man. He was found between runways closely followed by six soldiers, all of whom got on board with him. The tower operator then asked us if we would do him a big favor and try to pick up his wife and children, saying he would stay behind until his "last dying breath." I couldn't refuse a request like that under the circumstances, so Olson and Coalson, who had more room, affected a rendezvous, and picked up a group of people, which fortunately included the tower operator's family.

By this time, we were at minimum fuel and had to leave for Cu-Lao Re Island. After almost five hours in the Da Nang area, contact was finally made with our Volpar C-45. Apparently the customer in Nha Trang had a better use for it and had dispatched it on a courier run to Can Tho, south of Saigon, instead. It had just been released to support us! The pilot relayed that Mr. Francis was on a boat in the harbor and we were to pick him up. At this point in time, this was impossible due to our fuel state and passenger load. Since it appeared he was safe aboard a ship, we felt our job was done. We refueled at the island and arrived in Nha Trang about 9:30PM.

During this entire operation we were plagued by what seemed to be a lack of urgency on the part of the powers that be in Saigon. They probably couldn't believe what was happening. We couldn't either! However, what disturbed us more was the way the customers apparently viewed us. Although I thought I had been taken into their confidence, it turned out I was not made privy to the overall evacuation plan.

We were expected to provide all support to the customers, but our fate was apparently of no concern to them. Had we not been able to take off on the 28th, I wonder what support we would have gotten. I expect none.

On the brighter side, with few exceptions, all our personnel performed admirably. However, a small group of individuals went far beyond the normal call of duty. Without their efforts, we couldn't have come close to accomplishing what was done. They are Captains Terry Olson, Tony Coalson, Mechanics J. Gil, B. Pacariem and B. Phee. Well done!"

Back to Civilian Life and Helicopter Emergency Medical Services in the U.S.

"When we finally landed aboard the blue ridge on the night of April 29, we spent the next week or two at sea, finally arriving in Manilla and then on to Hong Kong for debrief. I arrived home in Utah about a week later.

I believe I was completely burned out on flying and the sad outcome of all the evacuations. It was about six years later (1981) that one of my pilots, Frank Stergar, who had followed me to Utah ended up talking me into visiting the army reserve unit that was based at the Salt Lake City airport. They were flying UH1 helicopters and a King Air. The marine reserves had no air wing in Utah. The army unit seemed to have a good operation and gave me a good sales pitch. I wound up being the old guy who kind of knew what he was doing. I had over 15,000 hours by then and did a lot of instructing for them. It was a good group. We were just down the ramp from Key Airlines which had the contract with the University of Utah flying a Bell 1-1 and 1-3. They approached me about flying for them. The idea intrigued me and sounded like something worthwhile to do.

I was with them for about a year or so. They were not a good outfit, but I did not have to deal with management very often, so I did not mind. The terrain and weather were similar to Laos except for the cold. It had its challenging moments but compared to flying in Laos it was not a problem for me. I must admit that I did a lot of things that I probably shouldn't have but it was not uncomfortable for me. However, I do clearly remember one winter afternoon there was a fast-moving front moving in and snow was falling. A flight call came in and the chief flight nurse came up to me and said we had a flight. I told her that the weather was not suitable at that moment, and we couldn't go. She looked at me and said, "but you have to go!" I demurred and told her it wasn't going to happen. Twenty minutes later, the snow stopped, and we went with no problem. But that was the attitude from medical personnel in those days who did not understand the risks and reason for weather minimums while most of the pilots were ex-Viet Nam veterans and comfortable with risk-taking. Not a good combination for Go No-Go decisions, especially with the added pressure of patient survival if not moved to a higher level of care.

I would go out on some flights that were pretty "tight," but I was not uncomfortable. There were times I would have to tell the crews not to talk about certain flights because it might put pressure on the other pilots to try to do the same thing. I will tell you that heading east out of Salt Lake City over the mountains at night in any weather with no navigational gear was challenging. Sometimes, I would flash the landing light and discover we were in the clouds.

Living conditions were far better than in Viet Nam, of course. Most of our medical transports in Viet Nam were last minute situations and consisted of simply landing at the sites and they would literally throw the bodies in the floor, particularly if they were under fire. The flight mechanic would do what he could but had no medical training.

After a few years with Key Airlines, who had the contract with the University for about 20 years, their contract came up for renewal. Air Methods was the only other bidder. At that time, the only hospital program Air Methods had under contract was in Grand Junction, CO. I really had no desire to go to work for someone else and knew nothing about Air Methods. I told their chief pilot that I had no interest and would be on my way if Air Methods was awarded the contract. But Roy Morgan, the CEO, tracked me down and I was so impressed with him that I finally said yes. I never regretted it. It was a year or two later that Roy twisted my arm again, asking me to go to Denver as the Director of Operations."

Summary

Marius's amazing and exciting account of his military experience culminates in the infancy of U.S. civilian air medical transport in the early 1980s. His invaluable insight and honesty are reflected in his words: "That was the attitude from medical personnel in those days, who did not understand the risks and reason for weather minimums while most of the pilots were ex-Viet Nam veterans and comfortable with risk-taking. Not a good combination for Go No-Go decision-making, especially with the added pressure of patient survival if not moved to a higher level of care."

In the early 1980s, when this part of Marius's career began there were only about 20 "programs". When we refer to programs in the next two chapters, these were hospitals (usually trauma centers) contracting with a helicopter FAA Part 135 operator to supply aircraft, pilots and maintenance based at the hospital. Helicopter medical transport is a much newer concept since airplanes had been used for many decades to transport patients, especially in rural areas.

In Chapter Three, Russ Spray will describe the aviation operator and business component of air medical transport, when it began and how it developed.

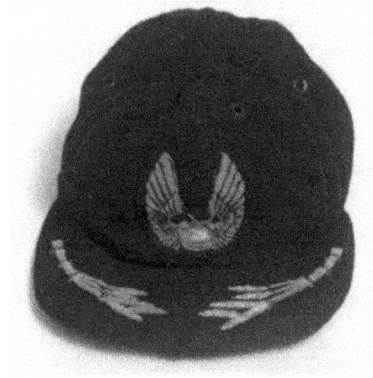

Post note: Sadly, Marius Burke passed away on October 29, 2020 at the age of 83 in Merritt Island, FL where he resided with his wife, Vinetra.

References

1. Cates, A. (2011). *Honor Denied: The Truth about Air America and the CIA*. Bloomington, IN: *iUniverse LLC*.
2. Glenn, M. (2021) 'It is not right': bill offers hope that flyers of CIA's Air America will finally win recognition. *Washington Times*. retrieved from: https://grothman.house.gov/news/documentsingle.aspx?DocumentID=2069.
3. Burke, M. (1989) Part 1 Danang Evacuation. *Air America*. 6(4). retrieved from: https://www.air-america.org/articles/evacuation-of-saigon-by-marius-burke.html.

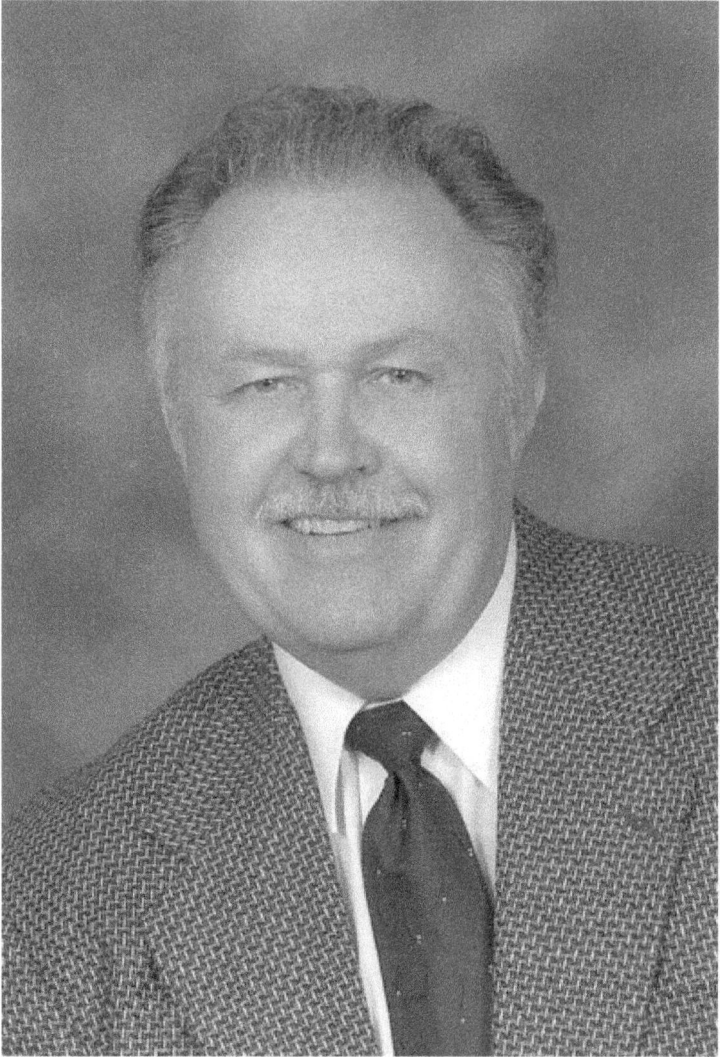

James Russell Spray

Chapter Three

James Russell Spray, Business Leader

James Russell (Russ) Spray was a "self-starter" long before most of us understand what we are supposed to be or do with our lives. Growing up in Southern California, Russ was surrounded by the aerospace and entertainment industries.

Russ's Uncle Jim was a flight navigator and a member of one of the original flight teams for TWA under the direction and ownership of Howard Hughes. When Uncle Jim visited, he would fascinate Russ with tales of flying and his travel adventures around the world.

The ever-adventurous Uncle Jim would eventually be assigned as a TWA instructor to Cairo, Egypt to assist in the joint-venture development of Saudi Arabian Airlines. Five years later, he left TWA to join Bill Lear in the development and introduction of the Lear Jet. After a brief stint wandering the world as a merchant marine navigator, Uncle Jim migrated back to Southern California to work for Pacific Airmotive Corporation located at Hollywood-Burbank Airport as an avionics/electrical engineer.

In the meantime, when Russ was just fifteen years old, his father had a severe stoke. His father ran an upscale retail clothing business in the entertainment district. Being an only child, Russ was forced to drop out of school to run the family business. This was not to be a normal care-free teenage life for Russ, but he was able to run the business until it could be sold several years later to provide a source of retirement for his parents.

Beginning a career in aviation

One afternoon, Uncle Jim stopped by the clothing store for a visit and suggested that Russ meet him at Pacific Airmotive that was opening a Pac Aero division focused on aircraft sales and flight training. It was during this visit that Russ was introduced to aviation and a career that would carry him throughout his life. Arriving at the Pac Aero Grand Opening, Russ noticed a small sign on the reception desk offering introductory helicopter rides on a Hughes 300 helicopter for $5.00. Russ's demonstrator pilot was Lauretta Foy, a former Women's Air Force Service Pilot (WASP) and an original Whirly Girl. Russ was fascinated by helicopters and Lauretta was intrigued by the young teenager's passion to fly. She became his first instructor and a second mother to him until her death at age ninety-one in 2004.

By age seventeen, Russ had attained his helicopter private pilot's license. He realized he was too young for most employers. He needed a commerical pilot license to earn a living flying helicopters but eighteen was the legal minimum age to fly commercially. The new General Manager of Pac Aero was Ralph Sharch - an old barnstormer. Ralph offered Russ an opportunity to become a ground instructor since it was possible to attain the Instrument Ground Instructor Rating without an age requirement. By age 18, Russ was appointed the Los Angeles Regional Area CAA/FAA Simulator Examiner for non-scheduled airlines operating in and out of the Southern California District.

Russ wasted no time to achieve his goals in aviation. On his 18th birthday, he tested and received his Commercial Pilot-Helicopter Rating along with his Certified Flight Instructor-Helicopter Rating on the same day. Colonel Hawk, the Director of the Flight Standards District Office at the Van Nuys Airport, tested Russ himself. It was Colonel Hawk's strong conviction that no one under the age of 21 should be operating commercial aircraft. But after eleven hours of testing that day, he had to concede that Russ met all the qualifications. Their friendship developed that day and continued throughout Russ's time in California.

While working for Pac Aero, Russ built flight hours trading instruction time on the helicopter for time on the airplanes with some of the older Pac Aero pilots - an opportunity that would raise questions from Colonel Hawk. How could Russ sign-off several students for their Commercial Check Rides only two weeks after Russ received his own license, he asked? Fortunately, after some hard chastising, the Colonel grinned and wished Russ a safe and successful career and complimented him on the knowledge and skills reflected by his students' recent check-rides.

During his tenure at Pac Aero, Russ was assigned as a fixed wing and helicopter instructor pilot and continued to pursue his helicopter experience providing helicopter support for VIP transports, electronic news gathering, aerial photography and highway and railroad construction surveying and support. His primary clients included the Associated Press, KNBC-Los Angeles, Warner Bros. Studios and Walt Disney Productions. Russ provided the only civil aerial photography over the 1965 Watts' Riots and conducted numerous VIP and flight photography missions. One of those assignments was to cover the opening of the new Matterhorn ride at Disneyland in Anaheim. The filming required Russ to maneuver his helicopter at a low altitude directly over the park resulting in a visitor complaint being filed with the FAA. The complaint was verified, but the FAA did not pursue further investigation once they learned the flight was ordered by Mr. Disney himself. Instead, Russ was counseled to pre-warn the FAA when performing such flights so they could be prepared to address any public concerns.

In the Fall of 1965, the War in Vietnam was beginning to escalate. Several of Russ's helicopter students were recruited to instruct for the US Military (Army, Air Force and Marines) and began relocating to Camp Wolters, Texas and Fort Rucker, Alabama. One evening while at home with his parents, Russ received a call from two of his current helicopter students. The students were excited to tell Russ that they had been accepted for interview with the defense contractor, Southern Airways, for instructor positions at Camp Wolters in Mineral Wells, Texas. They wanted Russ to fly with them in a rented plane and sign them off for the flight time to Texas. It was eight o'clock PM and when Russ asked when they wanted to go, they responded – now!!

The trip turned out to be quite a memorable night as Russ recalled. Crossing the Phoenix VOR at 1:00 AM, Russ reached down to switch the fuel tanks when the engine quit. Russ tried in vain to restart the engine but to no avail. Fortunately, there was just enough altitude to perform Russ's and his students' first dead-stick landing to Sky

Harbor Airport. The jolt of the touchdown freed an air block in the new selector valve allowing the engine to restart. They taxied the little aircraft to the terminal for a maintenance check and additional fuel resuming the flight for Texas without further incident. Incidentally, it was later determined that this new model aircraft had a defect in the fuel selector valve that was later modified but not before several accidents occurred.

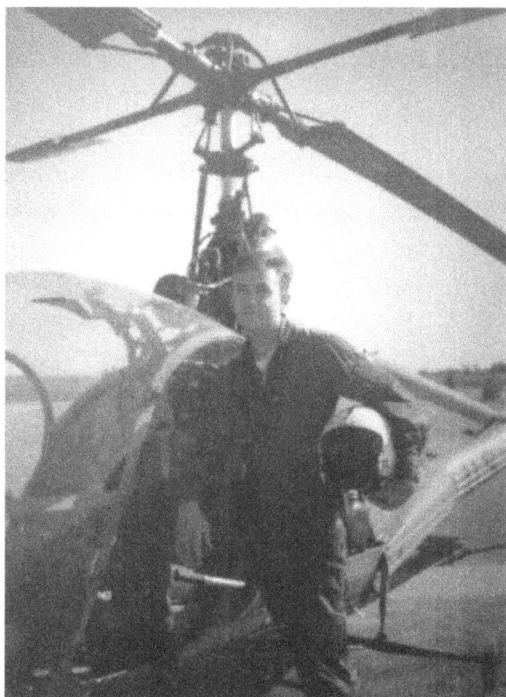

Russ at Fort Wolters in 1966

As the sun rose over El Paso, they set course for the next refueling stop at Wink, Texas. Upon landing, they were greeted by the ten-year migration of thousands of tarantulas that covered everything in sight. After a very hurried refueling, they took off for Mineral Wells. Once they were airborne, Russ climbed to the back of the airplane for a nap as he had been up all night. Both pilots were commercial-rated, and Russ felt comfortable leaving the last leg of the trip to them, instructing them to wake him up prior to landing. Somewhere over West Texas, a slight gust of wind caused Russ to awaken only to realize the aircraft was in a slow downward spiral. Both students were asleep at the controls! They were able to recover and reach their destination, but the experience left a lasting impression. For years following the incident, Russ could not bring himself to sleep on any airplane including as a passenger on airlines.

During the students' interviews at the Southern Airways' Camp Wolters Headquarters, Russ was approached by the Director of Training who wanted to meet the nineteen-year-old kid who was the instructor of the middle-aged pilots he had just hired. Returning to

California, Russ received numerous requests to join the Southern Airways team and he subsequently decided to relocate to Camp Wolters.

For the next seven years, Russ prepared beginning helicopter pilots for the Army, Air Force, Marines, and Allied Forces including students from Germany, Chile, Dominica, Iran, and Jordan. As the War in Vietnam continued to escalate, the operations at Camp Wolters grew and the base was soon commissioned as Fort Wolters with a General as Commandant.

The area surrounding Fort Wolters was adapted to imitate the topography of the areas in Vietnam with staging areas labeled Pleiku, Bin Hua, Hue, Da Nang, etc.

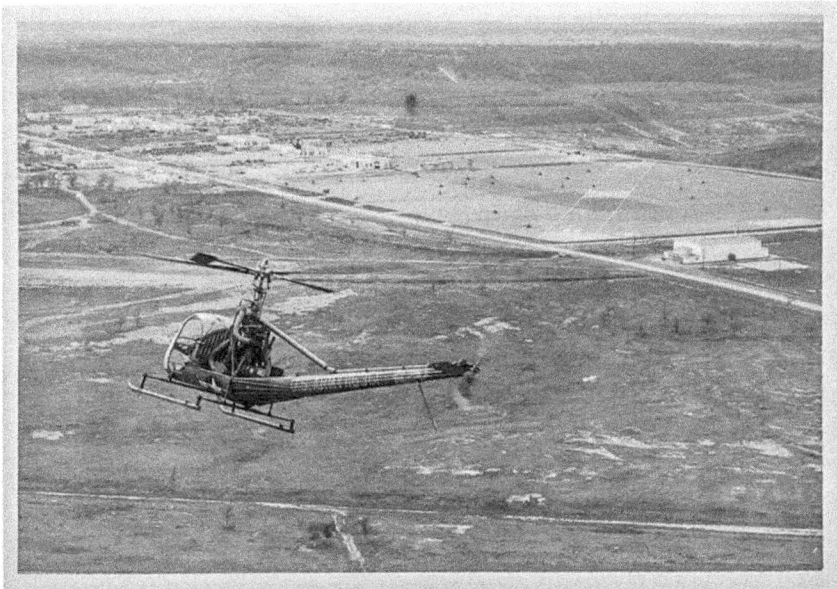

(Courtesy The Portal to Texas History) Pilots started training with the Hiller OH-23 at Fort Wolters' primary helicopter school.
http:\\airspacemag.com/history-of-flight/heroes-fort-wolters-180956245

Interestingly, the base was established in 1925 and was an important infantry-replacement training center with a troop capacity that reached 24,900 during World War II. Six months after the end of the war, the camp was deactivated. In 1951, it became the Wolters Air Force Base, and in 1956, it became a Primary Helicopter Center for the U.S. Army, renamed Fort Wolters in 1963. The Vietnam War increased the need for pilot training and at its highest level of activity, there were 1200 helicopters at this base. The base was deactivated in 1975, but memories of the training held there for both WWII infantry and helicopter training for the Vietnam War are still alive and well. Interesting to read all the comments from former trainees and families whose lives passed through this base over the decades.[1]

While Russ was instructing new recruits on OH-23D, the government instituted the draft and his number came up. Because Russ had to drop out of school at 15, he was not able to complete his high school education and due to a newly installed "no drop out" policy, the State of California would not honor the GED he received through correspondence at the University of California - Berkeley until he either joined a military service or reached age twenty-one. Therefore, he could not fly for the Army which required a minimum high school diploma or the Air Force, Navy and Coast Guard which each required two years of college at that time.

Russ hoped that his position as a military flight instructor would allow him to enlist in the Army's Warrant Officer Program. But even though he was actively training U.S. military officers at a military base, neither Russ nor the Warrant Officer Program Office in Washington could obtain a waiver to allow him to enter the flight program without the high school diploma. Russ continued to do flight instructing and was concerned about his future as a pilot when one summer afternoon he was called into the Commander's office. There he was met by Congressman Jim Wright who handed him a re-issued draft card with a Presidential deferment to continue the critical service of helicopter instruction.

Apparently the military, often accused of having no common sense, figured he was most needed as a flight instructor. Russ performed those critically needed flight training services from 1965 to 1972, training over 200 pilots for military duty during the height of the Vietnam War. Some student pilots were memorable and remained friends and acquaintances through the years. Several students worked under Russ's administration in later years in business endeavors.

Russ used any spare time during his military instructing years to concentrate on pursuing his formal education taking college level courses from Embry-Riddle on Base and traveling outside of the Fort to secure an Associate in Business degree at Weatherford College. The Associate Degree opened the door for Russ to seek his bachelor-degree and he began traveling the ninety-mile round trip each night after flight instructing to the University of Texas at Arlington. It was 1972 and Vietnam was winding down, so Russ took a voluntary separation and continued to pursue academic courses. Russ was always interested, since childhood, in physics and chemistry so he took pre-med and medical technology courses. Following an internship in Medical Technology, Russ received his Registry in Medical Technology from the American Society of Clinical Pathologists (ASCP).

Off to Iran

Russ's next full-time job was the evening Medical Laboratory Supervisor at All Saint's Hospital in Fort Worth. He became disenchanted with this work that often involved late night on-call duty. In the early morning hours before dawn, after an evening of hectic emergency calls, Russ grabbed a cup of coffee before heading home. With coffee in hand, he took an elevator to the top of the hospital for some quiet time and a view of the night sky across the Dallas-Fort Worth metroplex. Suddenly, a Huey helicopter flew by the window returning to the Bell Helicopter plant nearby. In his recent past, Russ was approached by the international team at Bell Helicopters to join them in support of new air cavalry training operations for a large-scale Foreign Military Sales program for the Shah of Iran. Russ took this fly-by as a sign and followed up with a direct call to his colleagues already positioned in Iran. In January of 1975, he was immediately hired and flown to Esfahan, Iran to return to the world of helicopters and the former ex-Vietnam military instructors with whom he had become close friends.

Esfahan was an ancient city surrounded by high mountains to the west where Alexander the Great had traversed to lay siege on Persepolis conquering the Persian Empire in the year 331 BC. Recalling history and observing the influence of the air cavalry experience of the US Military in Vietnam, Shah Reza Pahlavi decided to fortify the western front of mountain passes with mobile artillery supported by a force of helicopters. The Shah approached Bell Helicopters' top management to jointly develop a helicopter specifically capable of lifting a 105MM Howitzer cannon to a height of 9,000 feet MSL, operating in 95-degree F temperatures. With Iranian funding, the Bell 214 Heavy-Lift Helicopter was produced and placed into service to serve these specific needs.

The Iranian Mission was to create a strong military defense against the then Iraqi aggression. The Iranians lacked most of the skills required to support a sophisticated system of helicopters and airplanes and needed resources from the United States and its allies.

Prior to the close of the Vietnam War, Iran had sent a few student pilots for training at the military flight training centers in the U.S. For many of these students, the flight to the United States was their first experience in the air or in any mechanized form of transportation. The transition to a sophisticated turbine helicopter coupled with the language barrier proved difficult for many. So, upon arriving in Iran with the first detachment of instructors and air support personnel, Bell Helicopters representatives discovered a large fleet of Government of Iran (GOI) aircraft laying idle and unairworthy. Iran possessed a very limited supply of technically qualified citizens to staff their flight and maintenance needs. Therefore, a large recruitment effort was implemented to bring U.S. military experienced personnel to Iran to assure program success.

In addition, the GOI began a series of recruitment efforts within the towns and villages and even among the nomadic desert tribes of Iran to recruit adequate candidates for training.

The years in Iran proved both challenging and rewarding. Within the first year of arriving, Russ was promoted to Flight Commander and given the responsibility to manage a squadron of instructor pilots and control the training at GOI provided airfields, working with Iranian contractors and military personnel.

As the years passed, more and more foreign nationals, especially U.S. military and civilian personnel, entered Iran for military and commercial development. The population of these workers and their families grew from a few hundred to over 14,000. It soon became apparent that the local medical services were not adequate for this growing family. To retain employees, a higher level of medical care was essential. Russ was asked to take a brief sabbatical from his flight duties to help establish an American Clinic capable of handling emergent and family medical care. In conjunction with the Government of Iran (GOI) and Bell Helicopters, Russ was able to equip, staff and provision a small clinic on the outskirts of the city. This clinic remained in service until the civil revolution in 1979 forced closure and withdrawal of the clinic's staff.

Resuming his Flight Command, Russ continued supervising the training of GOI student pilots concluding his command with over 47,000 accident-free flying hours. As the years passed in Iran, Russ would occasionally return to the U.S. and Bell Headquarters in Fort Worth concluding with R & R, family visits and resupply, then back to his duties in Esfahan. On his last return trip to Esfahan, Russ observed the beginning of political unrest and the commencement of what was to become known as the Iranian Revolution. Within a brief six months of arriving back to Iran, the Revolution was on full-scale. U.S. military and embassy personnel were ordered to evacuate. By December 1978, the Iranian airspace was sealed by the Revolutionary Forces. Russ and the remaining forty-three employees and their families were evacuated in late January 1979 at 4:00 AM from a desert airfield back to the U.S. through Ankara, Turkey on a civilian volunteer-staffed airplane supplied by Pan Am.

New direction

Having escaped Iran with suitcase in hand, Russ returned to Fort Worth to plan his future and next of life's adventures. Taking time out to visit some friends and former employees, Russ stopped in Houston and was provided a tour at what became the second hospital-based helicopter EMS program in the U.S., Hermann Life Flight. It was at that moment that all of Russ's love and passions for medicine and aviation came together and he was determined to be a part of expanding the concept into a national network of air medical transport services for all of America's citizens.

Russ applied and was accepted for employment at the newly incorporated Air Medical Services located in Houston, Texas. This was a division of the Provo, Utah-based Rocky Mountain Helicopters, Inc. (RMH). At the time, RMH was the third largest helicopter company in the US and the largest supplier of helicopters supporting land-based seismic oil exploration and production services along with utility and motion picture support.

Quite by accident, while expanding shale oil exploration across the Rocky Mountains, RMH acquired Olympic Helicopters. This company had been contracted by St. Anthony's Hospital in Denver for transport with their medical teams to the nearby ski resorts in anticipation of the 1976 Winter Olympics. Although the Winter Olympics did not happen for Denver that year, the concept of using the helicopter with the hospital medical teams remained and was expanded to the inner-city needs.

While continuing its contract obligations to provide Helicopter Emergency Medical Services (HEMS) to St. Anthony Hospital, RMH was approached by Hermann Hospital administrators, its dynamic trauma surgeon, Dr. Red Duke, and Whitey Martin, Rescue Chief of the Houston Fire Department. They wanted a contract to provide helicopter services for a new urban program for the City of Houston. It was 1976, a few years before Russ evacuated from Iran. Chief Martin had a problem transporting his critical patients from the outlying areas surrounding Houston to the Texas Medical Center of Hospitals located inside the beltway. Calling it the "Denver Experiment," Chief Martin first went to the city with a request for a helicopter but was immediately rejected. Undeterred, Chief Martin went to a then-struggling Hermann Hospital and approached Bill Greene, Hermann's Administrator with a proposition: "You get me a helicopter and I will provide you with my patients." Bill accepted the concept of using helicopters to save lives was not just for mountainous areas, outlying highways and rural America but the services could also be applied to urban America.

In fact, in 1968, prior to the hospital-based Denver Flight for Life and Houston Life Flight programs, an experimental military project was developed in the southeast U.S. with limited success. Almost simultaneously a Children's Neonatal Transport program was created using an on-demand chartered helicopter in San Bernardino California.

In 1978, with the hiring of John Self, originally the Marketing Director for Hermann Life Flight, and with the blessings of Marguerite Badger, Program Director of Life Flight, Aviation Medical Services began a systematic campaign to replicate the Life Flight model at other trauma centers around the country. Within the next two

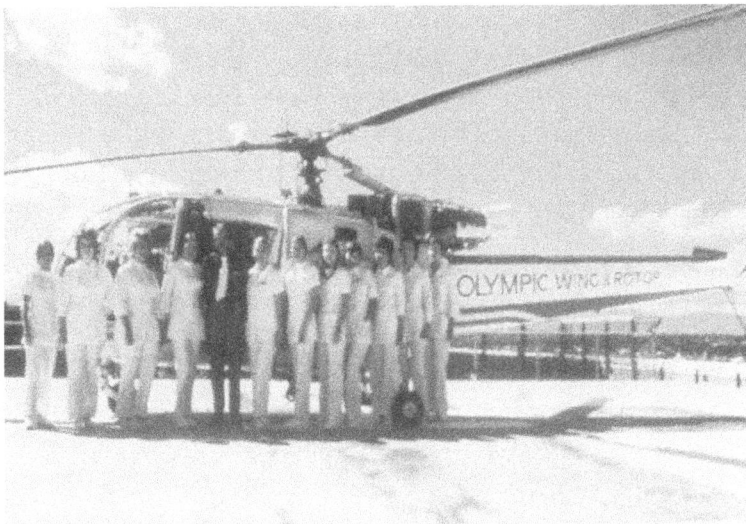

Dr. Boyd Bigelow and flight nurses from St. Anthony Hospital pictured here in 1972 with the Alouette leased from Olympic Wing and Rotor, the company set up to serve the 1976 Olympics in Colorado.

years, hospital-based helicopter programs were developed at Baptist Hospital, Pensacola, followed by Allegheny General Hospital in Pittsburgh, St. Joseph Hospital in Kansas City, Emmanuel Hospital in Portland, and Good Samaritan Hospital in Phoenix.

Shortly after joining Aviation Medical Services in February 1979, Russ was asked to transfer from Hermann Hospital and proceed to a new start-up program at St. Joseph Hospital in Omaha, Nebraska. Russ's level of experience and background in aviation and medicine along with a strong business experience and background made this new entity of air medicine the perfect fit for him.

Until 1980, RMH found little competition for its air medical services. Prior to this time most commercial helicopter services were devoted to oil exploration and production both on land and sea. Following Russ's escape from Iran and the pursuing Iranian Revolution, the Organization of Petroleum Countries (OPEC) was founded. This led to an increased oil production abroad and a price war that resulted in the closing of many of the domestic fields within the U.S. and a dramatic reduction in helicopter activity. So, RMH was not a lone FAA Part 135 provider for very long.

More and more aviation operators saw opportunities for contracts with hospitals in the early 1980s. Helicopter manufacturers also needed alternative markets for their drooping aircraft sales, and this had a dramatic effect on the marketing and development of helicopter services for the medical industry, electronic news gathering and a newly developing aerial law enforcement market.

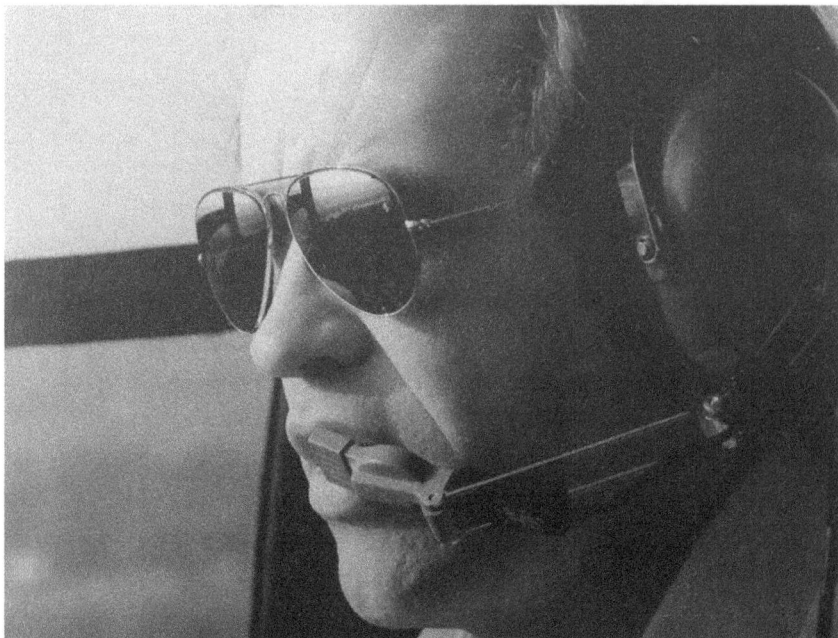

Flying at the start of Russ's HAA career in 1980

Helicopter manufacturers initiate a new marketplace

A growing number of FAA Part 135 Operators (meaning legally certified under FAA rules to transport passengers) were in a desperate position to provide services they had available but saw declining along with the oil production needs. But, it was the helicopter manufacturers who initiated the recognition of new helicopter EMS possibilities through advertising and direct marketing. This alerted other operators to the new marketplace and the manufacturers followed up by supporting operators with incentives to stimulate development and competition.

Helicopter EMS (HEMS) continued to evolve and expand across the U.S. At the same time, hospitals were incentivized by government grants to develop trauma centers and they needed helicopters to be a flying billboard for their trauma systems. Aviation and medicine had a common purpose at the same time and space in history.

However, the path to HEMS success was neither easy nor inexpensive. For example, there was a great deal of expense and down-time in setting up a trauma center for major trauma. Achieving a Level I trauma center status as defined by the American College of Surgeons – Committee of Trauma (ACS-COT) requires surgeons to be present in the hospital or readily accessible, including trauma surgeons, orthopedic surgeons, and neurosurgeons. Major trauma is beyond the scope of practice of Emergency Departments, so surgeons and the trauma team that includes the lab, blood bank, X Ray, anesthesia, and nursing teams need to be available as well as a specially equipped trauma operating room. The helicopter also must be available 24/7 with pilots, medical teams standing by and a communications center that goes beyond the 911 centers that were developed for ground ambulance Emergency Medical Services. The technicians in the communications centers needed to accept requests for EMS in the field and needed additional training in radio terminology for the medical and aviation disciplines – each with their own set of acronyms and terms that baffle most 911 communication centers.

These communicators were the link between the field requests, the helicopter and the hospital. The FAA 135 Operator was integral in providing additional training for the communications technicians. In addition, the FAA Operator needed to provide the appropriate aircraft as the topography in the U.S. varies and may require a helicopter for mountainous versus desert or coastal areas. Specific training for pilots conducting EMS responses was also developed. Most of the early pilots based at hospitals were ex-Vietnam pilots who likely had experience with life and death situations. The civilian HEMS culture was technically different from a war-time culture and the act of "completing the mission no matter what the consequences," led to risking weather "go or no-go" decisions and resulting in many weather-related crashes, as discussed in Chapter One. FAA 135 Operators have their challenges with managing pilots and mechanics at distant locations and setting policies that went beyond the FAA Part 135 regulations to keep crews and patients safe while performing in a time-sensitive environment. In addition, promoting a safety culture among disciplines with different skill sets and goals has always been a challenge.[2]

Russ was insightful, and he saw early on that helping to guide the relationship between aviation and medicine was important. He supported the start-up of a national trade organization called ASHBEAMS (American Society of Hospital-Based Emergency Air Medical Services). This organization held an initial meeting in Houston in 1980. Russ, representing RMH along with Howard Collett, the creator of *Hospital Aviation*[3] a monthly journal published by Aviation Hospital Consultants, sponsored the 1981 meeting in San Diego. There were approximately 30 attendees and an exhibit area made up of a few signs on a folding card table set in a hallway. These Air Medical Conferences continued each year to present times. ASHBEAMS is now AAMS – the Association of Air Medical Services. In 1987, there were 1000 attendees. Those numbers increase every year. In later years Russ went forward to reform and further develop the EMS Committee for the Helicopter Association International which he continued to Chair for over five years. Following this, he created the National EMS Operator's Forum operating today as the Air Medical Operators Association (AMOA).

In the 1980s Russ was busy developing new support delivery systems for RMH and moving contracts with hospital clients to longer terms (from 6 months to three to five-year agreements) to support the growing market demand for larger more expensive multi-turbine helicopters. At the same time, a number of states, in attempts to consolidate redundant medical services, sought to prevent the expansion of air medical services across state lines which might compete with existing local ambulance providers and state sponsored government agencies. The weapon of choice for the various states was the "Certificate of Need" and "Certificate of Convenience and Necessity" licensing. Initially this prevented an air ambulance operator from crossing state lines with patients which complicated regional rescues and referrals. Russ, through the national strength of RMH, was successful in campaigning to link HEMS with the Airline Deregulation Act allowing HEMS aircraft to be federally controlled and travel at-will across state lines.[4] This provided further growth for the industry through the 1980s and 1990s.

More and more demand for the FAA Part 135 Operators led to more operators entering the HEMS business. Competition started to become fierce as many newcomers in the business underbid hospital contracts just to get the contract making up on losses with support from the helicopter manufacturers seeking to broaden market competition. RMH was soon competing with Omniflight Helicopters, Air Methods, PHI, Evergreen, Keystone Helicopters, US Jets, EMS Helicopters, Pumpkin Air, Silver Star, and numerous others. Often contracts led to broken promises, and several of these new entities did not stay in business for long, often leaving hospitals without services until they could renegotiate with another Operator.

By the end of the 1990s, HEMS was well-established within the medical community as a valuable asset for patient care, and hospitals seeking trauma certification are required to have access to HEMS. The 1990s brought a new challenge for Russ and the HEMS Operators – the HMO. The Health Maintenance Organization concept began its life simultaneously on the East and West Coasts of America. It was a financial shift as the patient care and hospitals, once considered the profit centers, became the cost centers controlled by large insurance corporations.

Russ recognized that to continue to provide patient transport services in America, a new delivery concept had to emerge to satisfy the changing winds within American healthcare. He envisioned the day that hospitals under pressure from HMO's would be forced to dislodge their hospital-based and controlled HEMS along with other non-core activities. Thus, Russ set about to expand a concept of providing stand-alone services in which Rocky Mountain Helicopters (RMH) would offer to former customers the ability to continue aviation services with RMH and assume the once hospital-based responsibilities of onboard medical services and the final billing responsibility. LifeNet was born in Phoenix, Arizona in 1990 which has now become the basis of the community-based service model. Using this model, HEMS operators across the country have witnessed an aggressive expansion of HEMS services from 300 aircraft in 1990 to a projection of over 1250 HEMS aircraft by 2026.

Through its successes in HEMS, the RMH administration continued attempts to salvage a fleeting oil and gas utility market by expanding services into Aerologging, Fixed Base Operations,

Charter Jet Services, Commuter Airline Operations, Aerospace Manufacturing and five other business activities. Soon RMH over-extended its resources and cash flows. Under pressure from a major creditor and several financial backers, Russ was promoted to President and COO of the helicopter group. Russ immediately set about to rationalize several of the more unsuccessful business adventures. By the Fall of 1992, the Board of Directors of RMH requested that Russ replace the founder, Jim Burr, as Chairman of the Board

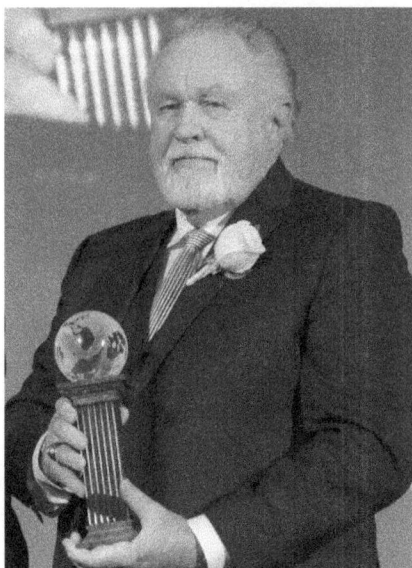

Russ received the Lifetime Achievement Award at HeliExpo in 2018

and Chief Executive Officer. Russ knew he needed more time to consolidate the operations to profitability, even for a time supporting payroll obligations with his personal assets. Acting as Chairman of the Board, Chief Operating Officer and Chief Financial Officer, Russ approached the Board for approval in 1993 to lead the company into a Chapter 11 Reorganization. RMH remained within Chapter 11 protection until 1995 when RMH was privatized with new capital from American Manufacturing and Dimeling, Schreiber and Park emerging as Rocky Mountain Holdings, LLC. In the succeeding years, RMH focused on its HEMS operations and doubled its size in revenue and profitability until its sale October 2002 to an acquisition by competitor, Air Methods Corporation (AMC), headquartered in Denver.

Summary

After several decades, Russ Spray ended his direct impact on HEMS in the U.S. but moved on to international business as the President and Chief Executive Officer for Turbomeca USA (recently renamed SAFRAN Helicopter Engines – USA), in charge of supporting North American manufacturing, repair and overhaul services for SAFRAN - one of Europe's largest aerospace manufacturers.

Today, there are major holding companies and big corporations driving the business of providing helicopter emergency medical services. There are fewer hospitals contracting with FAA Part 135 Operators. A few hospitals hold their own FAA Part 135 certificate, but some try this and fail because of the economies of scale. Larger companies have a cost advantage in keeping up with technology, offering back-up aircraft and decreased liability insurance premiums stretched out over larger fleets.

Typically, the larger corporate business managers – CEOs and financial officers are not fully acquainted with the business they are running. They see the bottom line – the costs and the reimbursement. They do not see the care providers that are impacting lives of patients and families with every transport. Russ was different because of his unique aviation and medical background and because he cared about the patients and crews. Russ knew it was important for the flight crews to have proper training, equipment, supplies and support from management. Russ was a recognized hands-on leader in the development of HEMS and his influence, vision and values are still reflected by the pilots and medical teams who dedicate their expertise and experience to the HEMS profession.

Chapter Four details the medical component and how the medical and aviation entities converged to form a cohesive profession, strewn with challenges and changes throughout its ever-evolving history.

References

1.   National War Museum. Fort Wolters. [Online.] Available at: https://www.nationalvnwarmuseum.org/development-plan/museum-themes/17-fort-wolters.html. (accessed November 1, 2021).

2.   Overton, J., Frazer, E. (2012). *Safety and Quality in Medical Transport Systems - Creating an Effective Culture*. Farnham, UK: Ashgate.

3.   Collett, H. 1985. An editorial opinion: hospitals and helicopters. *Hospital Aviation*. 4.(4).

4.   U.S. Congress. (1978). S. 2493 (95th): Airline Deregulation Act. [Online.] Available at: https://www.govtrack.us/congress/bills/95/s2493. (accessed November 1, 2020).

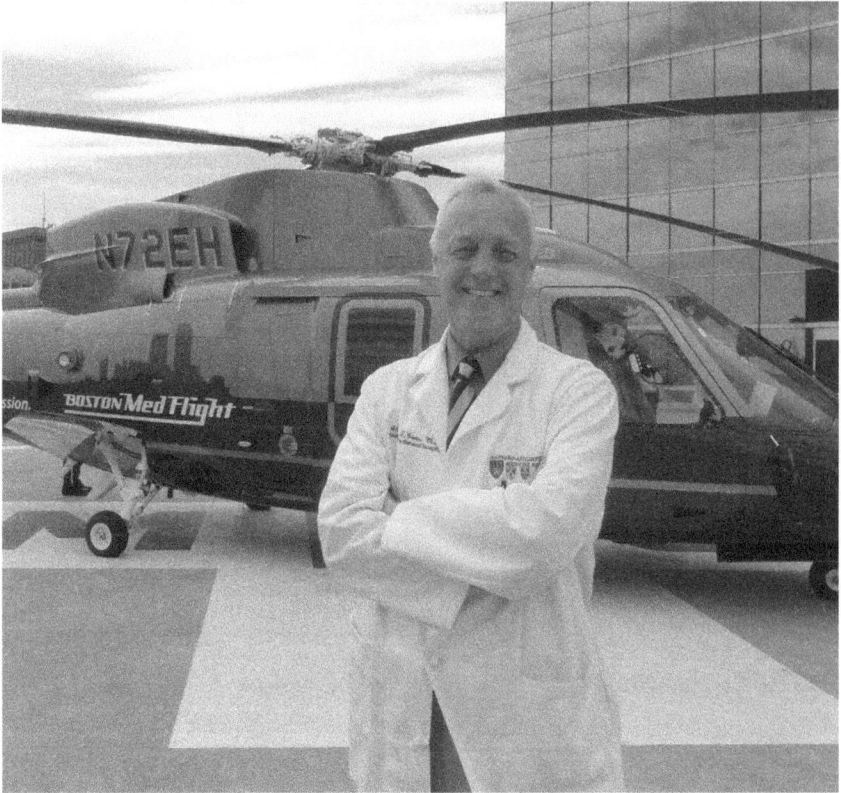

Dr. Alasdair Conn

Chapter four

Dr. Alasdair Conn - Emergency Medical Services and Trauma Centers

Background

As a registered nurse, graduating from nursing school in 1967, I started my career in an Emergency Department just as Trauma Centers were being formalized. Not only were trauma units a new concept for hospitals but Emergency Medical Services, as we know them today, did not start to develop until the 1960s. Of course, we can trace ambulances back to horse-drawn buggies in the Civil War. And there were several motorized ambulances seen in the early 1900s, but once the advent of automobiles led to more roads and travel, there was a more pressing need for updating transport practices, including emergency care for patients. For many decades, the hearses associated with funeral services would serve as the scoop and run vehicles with some early "rescue squads," but nothing was organized to standardize vehicles or develop medical practices to care for patients during transport.

Emergency Medical Transport has three major components: Transport vehicle; Provider education; and Communications. The Institute of Medicine's (IOM's) *"Accidental Death and Disability: The Neglected Disease of Modern Society" (1966)*[1], often referred to as the "White Paper," outlined the challenges and the need for an organized system. The IOM study found that more people died in auto accidents than died in Vietnam war up to 1965. Their findings included:

- Lack of a uniform law and standards
- Poor quality ambulances and equipment
- Lack of communications between EMS and hospitals
- No organized training for EMS personnel

Federal laws developed around this same time. The National Traffic and Motor Vehicle Safety Act (Public law 89-563) was passed in 1966 [2] followed by the Highway Safety Act (Public Law 89-564)[3]. These laws required that States develop safety programs to reduce accidents and deaths and provided financial assistance to States to accelerate safety programs. This also led to the development of the National Highway Traffic Safety Administration (NHTSA), originally under the Commerce Department until the Department of Transportation was developed in 1967.

The EMS Act of 1973[4] was the genesis of 911. In 1967, the Federal Communications Commission (FCC) started to meet with AT&T to establish this emergency contact number. They wanted a simple number that was easy to remember. In the early 1970s, the pilot program was tested in Alameda, CA. 911 would later be adopted by Canada and it has become the most recognized emergency number for any age group. There are numerous instances of small children dialing 911 for help, so it is known as a call for help from an early age.

The EMS Act also provided funding for the creation of more than 300 EMS systems across the U.S. The formal BLS and national Emergency Medical Technician (EMT) program also evolved from this act. Until the EMT training came along, ambulance attendees mostly depended on the American Red Cross First Aid Course which played a major role in treating injured in the military in WWI and continues till today training non-professionals and professionals in caring for those in crisis until medical professionals arrive.

In the 1960s, when I started working in an emergency department, the physicians were usually in general practice or surgeons who moonlighted for a shift in the ED. Before the 1970s, there were no residencies available for physicians to become certified as Emergency Physicians. The University of Cincinnati was the first to develop the Emergency Residency program in 1972. The American College of Emergency Physicians (ACEP), developed in 1968, offers board certification (FACEP) to physicians specializing in Emergency Medicine. Today, there are over 25,000 board certified emergency physicians practicing in the U.S.

The American College of Surgery (ACS), developed in the 1920s, also offers board certification - Fellow, American College of Surgeons (FACS). ACS currently has more than 82,000 members, including more than 6,600 Fellows in other countries, making it the largest organization of surgeons in the world.

After completing an approved residency in either surgery or emergency medicine, the physician must sit for boards approved by the American Council of Graduate Medical Education (ACGME). To carry the FACS or FACEP professional acronym behind their names, physicians must not only complete a residency in an approved program, but they must then be elected by their peers for their experience and significant contributions to the specialty. Health insurance companies recognize both boarded physicians or if not boarded, members of the ACS or ACEP to consider payments for treatment.

Physicians develop EMS basics

One of the most important skills taught to first responders is cardio-pulmonary resuscitation (CPR). The genesis of CPR is credited to Dr. Peter Safar (University of Pittsburgh) in the 1950s who allowed residents to ventilate him as they trialed the artificial manual breathing unit (ambu). Dr. Safar is known as the Father of Cardiopulmonary Resuscitation[5] and Dr. Knickerbocker, Dr. James Jude, and Dr. Kouwenhoven (Johns Hopkins University) are known as the Fathers of Compression[6]. In fact, Johns Hopkins took delivery of the very first defibrillator in May of 1959. It weighed about 45 pounds.

EMS further develops with the introduction of helicopters

The above are just highlights from the decades of progress that led to the pre-hospital care and transport we know today which continue to evolve. At the time, the public at large may not have been aware of these Acts and developing emergency response systems, but they knew TV shows like *Emergency!*, first aired in 1972. Many young people were inspired by John Gage and Roy DeSoto – the LA-based paramedics in the show. According to the book *Emergency! Behind the Scenes*[7], there were only twelve paramedic units in North America when the show began. By 1977, over 50% of all Americans were within ten minutes of an ambulance unit. *MASH*, another show that aired in 1972, became a classic based on the experiences of U.S. Army nurses and doctors at a Mobile Army Surgical Hospital (MASH) during the Korean War. The helicopter played an important role and was in the opening scene that told us exactly what this iconic show represented. It was done so well with a mix of humor and tragedy that the show lasted eleven years – longer than the Korean war itself.

One of the earliest and best-known experts bringing helicopter transport and trauma centers together was Dr. R. Adams Cowley, Father of Trauma Medicine. Dr. Cowley was affiliated with the University of Maryland Medical Center in Baltimore and the Shock Trauma Center (referred to simply as Shock Trauma) is named after Dr. Cowley who did extensive research of traumatic injuries in the 1950s culminating in the opening of Shock Trauma in 1959. Through his research, Dr. Cowley found that the quicker victims of blunt trauma were transported to the trauma center (where surgical intervention could be performed immediately) the better the patient's chances for survival. He coined the phrase describing this process as The Golden Hour - the hour immediately following a traumatic injury.[8] Working with the Maryland State Policy Aviation Division, Dr. Cowley was able to develop the first public service "civilian" helicopter transport service in 1969.

Dr. Alasdair Conn was a fellow at the University of Maryland Medical Center, working with Dr. Cowley during these trauma system and transport developmental years. His anecdotes about the process and personnel involved are fascinating. Dr. Conn is a pioneer and well-respected member of the American College of Surgeons – Committee on Trauma.

Dr. Alasdair Conn – *In his own words*

"I was born in Sheffield, England in 1948, post WWII. My father was a Professor of Physics at the University of Exeter. In my country, students go from high school to university based on your center of interest. I had an interest in molecular biology and biochemistry, but it was difficult to find a school with dual degrees so my degree in biochemistry led directly to continuing to medical school. I did my internship at the Royal Infirmary of Edinburgh. My last six months of clinical experience was in Spring 1971 on Ward 7 and 8 and my senior registrar was Bill Gill.

As I was completing my internship, Bill asked me to come to the U.S. where he was asked to help find staff for the new shock trauma center with Dr. R.A. Cowley in Baltimore. It was 1971 and I, along with three other new surgeons: Howard Champion, Bill Long, and John Sandiford traveled to Baltimore. We were starting a career in this new subspecialty of surgery called trauma as it was being studied and developed by Dr. Cowley and his associates at the University of Maryland Medical Center (UMMC). We always called Dr. Cowley "R.A."

R.A. was the professor of cardiovascular surgery and head of a twelve-bed unit a few years before I arrived at UMMC. Within this unit, there were two-beds reserved to study the hemodynamics of shock. Dr. Cowley was great friends with the Maryland State Police Aviation Division and his theory was that if rapid transport directly to surgical intervention worked in Vietnam - why would it not work here.

One evening, the Chairman of the Maryland House of Delegates was severely injured, with lower back pain and paralysis – fractures of L1 and L2. He was taken by ground ambulance to two different hospitals that were unable to manage him. Someone said: "Let's fly him to Dr. Cowley at Shock Trauma." After the patient was flown in, the governor, Marvin Mandel, came to visit. R.A. was never one to pass up an opportunity to solicit support for his shock trauma unit, so he took the governor aside and discussed how this concept of rapid transportation to the surgical unit would save lives and decrease disabilities from traumatic injuries for the public. At the time, the shock trauma unit had expanded to four beds, but R.A. needed more room, more beds, and more staff. Being part of a university system, shock trauma was not a top budget priority to administration.

In 1970, a representative from the University was asking for updates and budgeting resources for the University, and Shock Trauma was not at the top of his list. Frank Kelly, who was Chair of the Senate budget committee, supported Dr. Cowley's need for more funding. Frank Kelly was trying to put more money in the budget for the trauma unit but not getting anywhere with his "but Cowley is saving lives" speech. The Chancellor was emphasizing that the law school needed funding and was not agreeing. In exasperation, Kelly told the Chancellor that he could not fire him, but he could reduce his salary to $1.00 next year if the Chancellor did not agree to more funding for the trauma unit. The support was appreciated but this put R.A. at war with the University.

In short order, Cowley received an executive decree from the University stating that they were closing the trauma unit and all the expected funding would not go to shock trauma but would go to the Department of Surgery.

But Cowley's former politicking with the Governor paid off. He called the Governor to relate the University's intention to close the trauma unit. The governor responded with an Executive Order that bypassed the trauma unit from the university hierarchy with Cowley now reporting to the governor. The shock trauma budget would come directly out of the State.

When I and my three mates from England arrived, the Critical Care Resuscitation Unit (CCRU) at the University of Maryland Medical Center was arranged like a spaceship. There were beds on both sides and the physicians and nurses stood in the middle and could see all the monitors surrounding them. This patient reception unit was on the 4th floor. The ground floor was the waiting area for families, the 2nd floor was the trauma operating rooms (ORs). The third floor housed the dedicated labs. Patients were brought in by

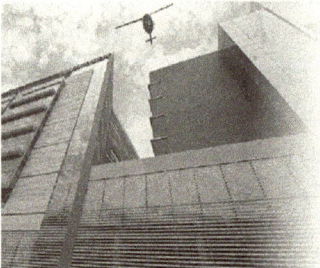

R. Adams
Cowley Shock
Trauma Center

Baltimore, MD

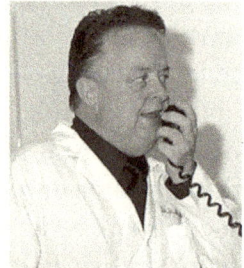

source: https://www.google.com/search?q=dr+r+radams+cowley

84

ground and air, arriving by the elevators. Those elevators were at the back entrance to the hospital. Space in large cities is always scarce, especially for landing helicopters. The helicopter landed on top of a parking deck about a block away. An ambulance met the helicopter and drove down a winding parking deck to the street below and then drove through the waste disposal dumpsters at the back entrance of the hospital to reach the shock trauma elevators.

Syscom, the communications center, at first was a 12X12 room. We had a hot line to the State police helicopters. In addition to the pilot, there was one police officer on board who had EMT training. Anytime there was a scene call, they would call in on the yellow phone in the trauma unit. I remember one time - a patient in Bed #9 asked me why the staff seemed to get so excited when the yellow phone rang, especially since it meant someone was injured. I explained that we were glad that we could save another life and we liked to excel at what we do – so more patients gave us the opportunity and experience to be our best.

These earlier days in civilian aviation did not have the weather reporting systems or GPS navigation tools that are available today. I wondered what it was like during a transport, so I did go along on a request to Prince George's County. We followed headlights on the road – then we would suddenly go up as the pilot said "WIRES" to let us know why we suddenly went nose up. We would go about 100 yds, circle around to find the headlights, and then continue to the red lights at the accident location.

I was at Shock Trauma from late September 1972 until June 1974. When I left England, my superiors in Edinburgh told me they would keep my job open for a year. They thought I would be back. I wanted to stay in the U.S., but I was more concerned about my father's opinion. He surprised me. My father was a physicist, who went to Cambridge, and was involved in putting radar into airplanes at the end of WWII. After the war. he told me he had been invited to be Chairman for the Dept. of Physics at the University of Wisconsin. But he declined. He said he made the wrong decision in not going to the U.S. and regretted it. He supported my decision to stay in the States saying, "You need to look forward, not back."

From Shock Trauma, I applied to Duke University Hospital and was accepted. The Chair of the Dept. of Surgery was Dr. David Sabiston, Jr. who wrote the *Textbook of Surgery*[9] and was a legendary figure in American medicine. He only took in 12 students and there was a 2nd year position open. Dr. Sabiston offered me that position due to my 1.5 years at Shock Trauma. However, the student who was leaving decided to stay, so my offer was back down to 1st year resident. At the same time, I also received an acceptance from the University of Toronto. Graduating from this program was acceptable worldwide so I chose the University of Toronto. I finished there in 1978 as a general surgeon, boarded in Canada and America.

From there I went back to Shock Trauma. When R.A. asked me to come back, he said I needed to sign the contract. I said I needed to think about it and commented that the contract did not have any numbers. He said, "Don't worry about it – we will fill that in later." The next day I sent R.A. a telegram saying, "Yes." The following day, I was in surgery when the hospital porter knocked on the door stating he had an urgent telegram for me. The message was simply: "Fantastic - R.A. Cowley."

In 1978, I was now a trauma attending and the unit had expanded. We had our own orthopedic and neurosurgical groups covering 24/7 along with plastic surgery. Since this was an independent unit, we were not limited to coverage from the University. We also had surgeons from Johns Hopkins Hospital, a renowned medical center and research facility in Baltimore.

I became great friends with the pilots and EMTs and they wanted to become EMT Intermediates (EMTIs) meaning they could do invasive skills like starting intravenous lines (IVs). They made me medical director of the aviation program of the MD State Police. There were no patient simulators back then, so my arms were the practice sites for the EMTs to develop their IV skills. Then they wanted to become paramedics as this was becoming the recognized standard of care for Advanced Life Support (ALS). There was no national paramedic curriculum at that time, so every state had its own course. We put a law into Maryland for a state paramedic program and this meant there needed to be a state medical director. I was asked to fill that role.

By that time, R.A. was head of the EMT program because nobody wanted it. In many States, EMTs were part of the fire department. The fire department was able to request more funding for EMTs, but the EMS part of their budget was secondary to Fire wants and needs. Fire was always the primary focus, so this was a challenge. As the State Medical Director, I ran into friction from the fire service because we now had a state paramedic exam. The fire dept. said just give us the test and we will pass it out, but I wanted to have exams like those of physicians and nurses – timed and independent testing. R.A. then developed an oversight board with all the fire chiefs. We were one of the first to develop state-wide EMT and paramedic criteria (BLS and ALS) and this became so political that it was time for me to leave. An opportunity came up in Boston.

Prior to my arrival in Boston, Dr. Lenworth Jacobs was director of the ED at the Boston City Hospital. At that time, there were Basic EMTs in Boston, but Len wanted to upgrade them to paramedics, and he got a law passed to develop the paramedic program in Boston. Medical control is the Emergency Dept. physician or appointee who gives direction to paramedic in the field in real time. These paramedics got medical control from the Boston City Hospital but what was happening was not acceptable to the major medical facilities in Boston. The paramedics would get the medical direction and drive past closer hospitals to go to Boston City Hospital. Soon other hospitals petitioned to have medical control. Intense rivalry ensued between the other hospitals and Boston City Hospital. Massachusetts General Hospital (the largest teaching hospital of Harvard Medical School) was the last hospital to get medical control approved.

After a few years, Len said: "Now let's get a helicopter!" And he was wise. The state had a Certificate of Need (CON) process and so he went to UMass Memorial in Worcester (a state supported system) to get support for a statewide system with nurses and paramedics on helicopters at UMass and in Boston at Boston City Hospital. These were 2 separate applications – one for UMass and the other Boston City Hospital. Many other hospitals in Boston lobbied against the proposal and the Commonwealth was informed that if permission was given to an individual hospital there would be multiple applications from many hospitals for the same resource. The State approved UMass in Worcester but would not approve Boston City Hospital and said they required a consortium of hospitals for the city of Boston. UMass began flying and on July 14, 1984, they had a fatal accident. The pilot and physician died. The nurse was critically injured. The patient did fine and was transported by ground. The wife of the physician sued UMass and was awarded $40 million.

They continued flying after the accident, but they were not just flying trauma. They were flying cardiac and stroke patients and taking them back to Worcester. This really upset the Boston hospitals, so they formed a consortium as the State had required. To lead this process, they wanted the person selected to have trauma experience, knowledge of helicopters, legislative processes and never worked before in a Boston hospital so that there was no favoring one hospital over another. My experience fit these requirements and I was selected. This is why I moved to Boston in 1985. The agreement for the consortium was that all the hospitals would chip in and the Boston City Hospital agreed to provide the accommodations and the communications. I was hired to do 50% administrative and 50% emergency surgery care. They were going to lease a BK117 helicopter through Keystone Helicopters, in West Chester, PA.

In setting up the medical teams, I had to take a nurse from each hospital to be politically correct. There were very few nurses at that time who had any transport much less flight transport experience. At the time I called around to other programs that were using BK117s, and I contacted Mary Hart. Mary was a flight nurse who had started the Portland, OR and CALSTAR in CA programs. She had all the training put together. She was asked for a two-year commitment and that is what she gave us. Mary was very tough but provided crew training that gave us an excellent start. She even made the flight uniforms for the crews.

I reported to the Board with representatives from all the hospitals. I asked about insurance – will they cover transport charges? Negotiations with third party payers had not been completed at the time of program implementation. Within the 1st year, we put in a bill that mandated that if you were flown and a physician said it was appropriate, the insurers had to pay. When we went before the committee to introduce this bill, the first witness was a six-year-old

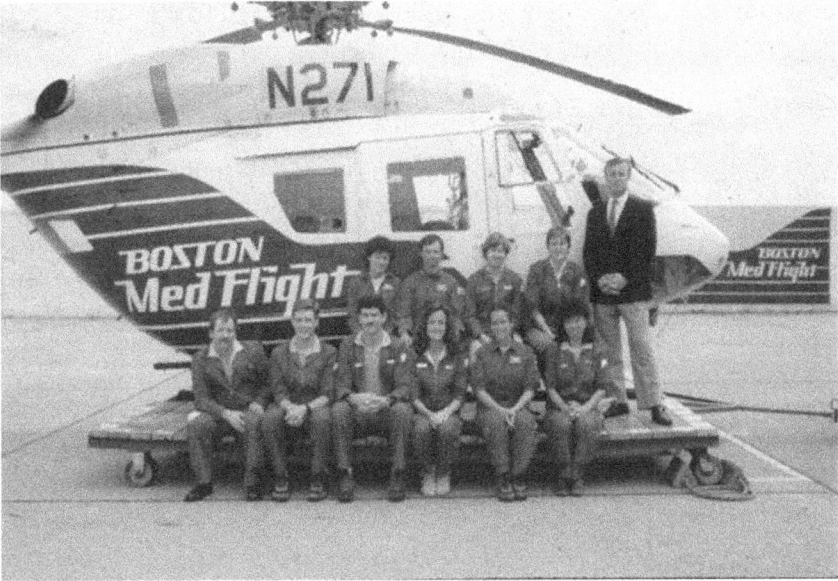

1989 Dr. Conn with flight crew

hit by a drunk driver and flown to the trauma center. Her father was a fire fighter, and they were on Cape Cod when this happened. The local hospital was not equipped to handle her injuries, so they needed to fly her to the Tufts New England Medical Center. She recovered very well and her testimony that began by saying: "the helicopter saved my life" was convincing.

After 2 hours of additional supporting testimony – only one insurer said it was too expensive and it was experimental. After much negotiation, we agreed to put the bill in abeyance because 3rd party payers agreed to put in about 2 million and the hospitals would kick in the rest.

Together with other programs in New England, we developed the New England Air Alliance that exists to today with programs sharing information, flight following, LZ protocols and backing each other up.

With computer aided dispatch platforms, we are able to share locations of aircraft so that the closest aircraft responds, or more than one available aircraft can be dispatched to multi-casualty incidents. Adult and pediatric patients go to the closest Level 1 Trauma center. The underlying premise is that rapid transport by helicopter is for those who are critically injured. If you are sick enough to be transported by helicopter, you will be transported to a Level I Trauma Center, not a Level II Trauma Center.

Trauma center designations

There have been several preventable deaths studies, testing Dr. Cowley's "Golden Hour" theory to verify rapid transport and treatment to a trauma center, where immediate surgical intervention is available, does impact outcomes. The best-known study was Dr. Don Trunkee and Dr. John West's preventable death study, published in 1979 and entitled "Systems of trauma care. A study of two counties." This study compared 90 cases of multiple trauma victims in Orange County, CA, who went to several local hospitals to 92 multi injured in San Francisco who went to a single trauma facility at San Francisco Hospital. They found that 30% of the deaths in Orange County were preventable while only one death in San Francisco was potentially preventable. These appalling results led to more studies to develop criteria to designate trauma centers in Orange County. Forty percent of the hospitals in the county applied and wanted to be a trauma center. R.A. was selected to evaluate the county's criteria for designating trauma centers, and he asked me to come along. The American College of Surgeons (ACS) was not involved at that time.

The county created their own criteria for designating hospitals as trauma centers. The main criteria required 24-hour in-house surgical, anesthesia CAT scans, labs, etc. capabilities. They designated 5 hospitals in Orange County located at geographic distances and that made sense. Forty hospitals applied. This was the beginning of the trauma center designation process.

Bob Heilig, from the EMS office in Orange County, asked if he could come back and see Shock Trauma in Baltimore, because he had never seen a functioning trauma center.

In the follow up Orange County studies, preventable deaths went down to 15% and then 5%.

Meanwhile in San Diego County, Dr. Steve Schackelford went through the same process. Their survival rate went down in their studies from 25% to less than 5%. So, the designation process began to take shape with little increase in resources – mostly reorganization. It was becoming apparent that this was a political process and there needed to be a more officially recognized designation process.

In Erie PA, there were two competing hospitals. One announced they would be the trauma center. They marketed heavily with local EMS and developed their own criteria. One of the criteria was that the hospital must have a surgical residency program which the other hospital did not have. So, the local EMS agency tried to designate the hospital with surgical residents as the trauma center. The other hospital challenged the local EMS agency and the Secretary of State in PA agreed stating no designations could occur until enabling state legislation was passed.

It was obvious to many that a national organization such as the American College of Surgeons - Committee on Trauma (ACS-COT) should be involved in this process. However, ACS is a professional organization and does not have the authority to dictate where a patient is required to go for specific types of care. Only a state can pass laws to direct a trauma patient past hospital facilities – not the county or town government agency. The state of Utah went a step further and was one of the first to pass legislation to designate trauma centers that included the process of calling in the ACS to verify the trauma center as being in compliance with the standards and criteria for the different Levels of Trauma Centers.

The ACS finally agreed to being part of verification - not the actual designator of trauma centers. The States designate and the ACS verifies. This gives the States the ability to say where the trauma patient should go based on designating trauma centers and based on the ACS criteria. Most States use the ACS criteria and legislation usually says something like, "Hospital facilities need to obtain and maintain verification by the ACS or another recognized body" and can apply for trauma designation after they obtain verification.

However, most States do not limit the number of trauma centers in a particular geographic area and that is why in Boston, we have five Level 1 adult trauma centers and three Level 1 pediatric trauma centers – probably too many. The ACS-CoT did add numbers to their verification process. For example, to be a Level 1 adult trauma center, you should admit 1,200 multiple trauma patients annually. But then is an elderly patient with a broken hip and a head laceration considered multi-trauma victim while a teen with similar injuries may not be? With endless variables, like age and coexisting conditions, it becomes difficult to define and differentiate.

We have learned some lessons along the way. After Orange County designated the 5 trauma centers, one of the hospitals said they no longer wanted to be a trauma center. The volumes were not there to financially support the number of personnel being paid to stand by for trauma cases. There was a part of the agreement that as a trauma center you need to have a 60-day cool down period so that other arrangements could be made. And you need to remain open for those 60 days. During this 60-day period, a patient came into this facility who needed surgical intervention, but they had to wait for the surgeon to come in. He was not standing by in the hospital as required. The patient died and the family sued. The county was not found at-fault, but the hospital was found liable because they did not abide by the rules.

Another learning point in the process of designation was an interesting lawsuit in Orange County.

There was a patient stabbed in Disneyland. A nurse on a go cart took the patient with multiple stab wounds to the community hospital a few blocks away. The family sued because, by trauma triage criteria, a patient with multiple stab wounds should have gone to the trauma center initially, not secondarily. This made an impression on EMS to think about the liability of not taking a multi-trauma patient to a trauma center.

In 1990, there was a Trauma Care Systems Planning and Development Act to improve emergency medical services and trauma care. The National Highway Traffic Safety Administration (NHTSA) was also active in contributing to trauma systems development. They stated they can prevent deaths by dealing with things before and at the time of the crash like speed limits, seat belts, helmets for motorcycle drivers, and appropriate more tax money to states to fix highways and enact these safety mandates.

The federal government can add dollars to a state and its highway safety funds to support such preventative measures and a small percentage of a several million-dollar annual awards is enough to persuade states to look at such enabling legislation."

Conclusion

In conclusion, I asked Dr. Conn where he thought helicopter EMS programs would be in the future. We discussed the increased number of independent helicopter services that result in increased competition, fewer flights because they are spread out over more services, and higher charges for patients. When flight volumes decline, the fixed costs of a helicopter and highly trained transport teams become less manageable. Dr. Conn felt that insurers were going to set the tone for acceptable charges.

There have also been several bills introduced to remove HEMS services from inclusion in the Airline Deregulation Act of 1978. There is a preemption clause in this act that prevents states from imposing economic regulation on the airline industry. States often argue that they have no control over how many helicopters penetrate their state because of this act. But this is a complicated issue that continues to weigh over the needs for HEMS services versus the number needed and who makes that decision.

There will be continual need for HEMS as community hospitals need assistance to get critically ill and injured patients to the major centers of excellence and trauma centers. There are also many rural areas that use HEMS for patients that need access to care even if they are not critical. A ground transport in rural areas may take too many hours and leave their coverage area with no ambulance for the next patient in need. Dr. Conn specifically felt the specialty care teams such as at pediatric and neonatal centers would continue to use helicopter transport for critically ill children and infants.

Technical advances like drones are already delivering organs to transplant recipient hospitals. Additionally, community paramedicine, also known as mobile integrated health and telemedicine are rapidly rising as alternatives to chronic and frequent 911 ambulance requests. These have shown to be cost saving and effective parts of healthcare to decrease the high costs of transport and hospital readmissions.

In summary, EMS, ground, and air, continue to evolve, expand, merge, and strive to meet the emergent and continual care needs of our communities through a dedicated and established workforce.

References

1. National Academy of Sciences. (1966). *Accidental death and disability: The neglected disease of modern society.* [Online.] Available at: https://www.ncbi.nlm.nih.gov/books/NBK222962/. (accessed July 1, 2020).
2. Wikipedia Foundation n.d. National traffic and motor vehicle safety act. (1966). [Online.] Available at: https://en.wikipedia.org/wiki/National_Traffic_and_Motor_Vehicle_Safety_Act (accessed July 2, 2020).
3. U.S. House of Representatives. (1966). The highway safety act of 1966. [Online.] Available at: https://history.house.gov/Historical-Highlights/1951-2000/The-Highway-Safety-Act-of-1966/ (accessed July 1, 2020).
4. 93rd Congress. (1973). Emergency medical services systems act. [Online.] Available at: https://www.congress.gov/bill/93rd-congress/senate-bill/2410. (accessed July 2, 1990).
5. PMC. Lenzer, J. (2003). Peter Josef Safar: The father of cardiopulmonary resuscitation. *NCBI Resources.* [Online.] Available at: https://www.ncbi.nlm.nih.gov/pmc/articles/PMC194106. (accessed July 1, 2020).
6. National EMS Museum. (2011). Johns Hopkins celebrates 50 years of CPR. [Online.] Available at: https://emsmuseum.org/collections/archives/defibrillators/1957-first-defibrillator. (accessed September 24, 2021)
7. Yokley, R. Sutherland, R. (2008). *Emergency! Behind the scene.* Sudbury, *MA. Jones and Bartlett Publishers.*
8. Edlich RF, Wish JR, Britt LD, Long WB. (2004). An organized approach to trauma care: legacy of R Adamas Cowley. *jllongtermeffmedimplants.* v14.i6.50.
9. Townsend, J. C. M., Beauchamp, R. D., Evers, B. M., & Mattox, K. L. (2016). *Sabiston textbook of surgery* (20th ed.). Elsevier - *Health Sciences Division.*

EPILOGUE

In my journey as the Executive Director of CAMTS, I have met many wonderful care providers, pilots, mechanics, and communicators – those who carry out the actual day-to-day work. I know that these front-line professionals are dedicated, caring and exceptional. Providing this service, however, has become big business and we have seen many changes over the past four decades. Hospital-based services are now in the minority. Private, independent for-profit companies provide most of the helicopter and fixed wing services today in the U.S. Many of these companies have adapted the CAMTS standardized processes and we currently have over 200 programs accredited.

But healthcare in the U.S. is tumultuous and this trickles down to medical transport. It is a challenge to support crews 24/7 to respond when needed; keep up with technology and training; and provide certificated aircraft and ambulances when the only income is from patients and patient insurance coverages. Medicare and Medicaid reimbursements are far below costs, and we cannot refuse to transport a patient with a life-threatening emergency, no matter the ability to pay.

When helicopter emergency medical services developed as part of hospital trauma systems, the helicopter costs were regarded as part of the overall inpatient charges. The helicopter was considered a flying billboard to bring patients into centers of excellence. But hospitals found that outsourcing the helicopter service to private companies was cost effective and they were still able to receive the patients. We have seen this trend continue and we have also seen consolidation and mergers of a few major aviation operators, providing nation-wide services.

Recently, I met someone who told me he was managing a medical helicopter service in a poor, small country with limited resources. The sponsor was a philanthropist who was interested in providing the most up-to-date aircraft and well-trained teams and they wanted to achieve accreditation. He described how the teams had to live behind fenced in areas and how his car had been shot at when traveling outside their protected area. I asked him "Why"? Why did his sponsor want to spend the time and effort on this endeavor? He said that for the sponsor, it wasn't a hobby or another tick on his philanthropic list. He felt he had the means to respond to a needed service. Also, both the sponsor and the crews really cared about the people and in many cases this was their only access to definitive care if they were seriously ill or injured.

This is where and why we started out – to care for those who are seriously ill or injured regardless of ethnicity, color, or ability to pay. My hope going forward is that we will continue to be true to this simple mission and that the values of big business do not overpower our practices and cause us to forget where we came from.

No one knows more about air medical services than Eileen Frazer. In The Emergence of Helicopters and Hospitals, she brings readers on the fascinating journey of how helicopters and their crews became lifesavers. Her story and those of medical and industry giants in medical transport reveal a history that will shape the future of air medical services

—Richard C. Hunt, MD, FACEP
Former Vice-Chair, Commission on Accreditation of
Medical Transport Services; Former Medical Director, EastCare;
and Former Director for Medical Preparedness Policy,
National Security Council Staff, The White House

I got chills reading this book because it took me back 42 years to my first exposure to helicopter EMS. As a young EMS system administrator in Eastern PA, working to put all the pieces of a regional EMS system together, I received a call one morning in 1980 from Dr. Michael Rhodes, an equally young, energetic, and persuasive Chief of Trauma from what was then the only trauma center in our region.

He told me to meet him in the parking lot of the hospital at high noon so he could show me another piece of the "EMS system puzzle" he was working on.

Shortly after I arrived, I heard the whop-whop of a massive green Vietnam-era HUEY helicopter on the horizon. I thought, "Oh my God no; he's never going to get a massive helicopter like that to land on our roadway." He told me to relax, hop in and "just absorb the concept."

He had the pilot, Lach Brown, take us all over the region. As we flew, Lach announced how long it took for us to traverse the region.

Just before we landed, "Dr. Mike" told me he would have a small, "sports car" medical helicopter, a Messerschmitt BO-105, on his landing pad within a year if I agreed to work with him on training, communications, and operational issues. I believed in him, pledged my full support and Mike Rhodes worked tirelessly to have his program up and running within a year.

Eileen Frazer was one of the amazing Medevac team members he recruited to make it all happen. Her book is a must read for all EMS personnel, particularly those who want to learn about what it took to make aeromedical EMS happen in the United States.

—A.J. Heightman, MPA, EMT-P
Editor-Emeritus *Journal of Emergency Medical Services (JEMS)*

One thing I have encountered in the past few years is the lack of "memory" of nurses, doctors and EMS personnel became involved in the transport of critically ill and injured patients. The Emergence of Helicopters and Hospitals provides a history of how helicopter transport became an integral part of patient care both from the field to the need for transport to specialty care. It also looks at the development of the importance of safe transport for both the patient and the caregivers.

I know all who are currently involved in patient transport need to read where we came from. I also hope that those of us who have moved on, take pride in what has been accomplished, especially through the dedication of the work of Eileen Frazer and her other authors.

—Renee Semonin Holleran, FNP-BC, RN-BC, CEN, CFRN, CTRN, (retired), CCRN (alumnus), PhD, FAEN Formally with University Air Care, Cincinnati Ohio and Life Flight, Salt Lake City, Utah

Eileen Frazer has spent her career striving to improve the quality and safety of air medical transportation in the U.S. and internationally. With her early career experience as a flight nurse in a helicopter transport program (HEMS) and subsequently in her role as the Executive Director of the Commission on Accreditation of Medical Transport Systems for over three decades, she tells the unique story of how air medical transport programs have evolved and their efforts to improve the outcomes of patient transport by air. Ms. Frazer is a highly respected international leader in air medical transport and in this text does a terrific job of sharing the important history of the evolution of helicopter transportation of our critically ill and injured citizens - a story that has not been told this completely by other authors or sources. This history will be interesting to those working in EMS, in all modes of patient transport and those working in critical care medicine.

—John Overton, Jr., MD, FACS
Former member of the CAMTS Board of Directors
Co-Editor of *Safety and Quality of Medical Transport Systems*

INDEX

A

accident - 7, 21, 25

Advanced Life Support - (ALS) - 86

Advanced Trauma Life Support (ATLS) - 10, 97

Air America - 6, 33, 34, 35, 37, 41, 56

Airline Deregulation Act of 1978 -73, 93

Air Medical Operators Association (AMOA) - 72

Air Medical Safety Committee - 5, 20, 27

Air Methods Corporation (AMC) - 74

Al Francis - 40, 42, 49

AMRM - 24

American College of Emergency Physicians (ACEP) - 23, 80, 81

American College of Surgeons - Committee on Trauma - 71, 81, 90, 91

Air Medical Resource Management (AMRM) - 15

American Council of Graduate Medical Education - 81

American Society of Hospital Based Emergency Air Medical Services (ASHBEAMS) - 20, 21, 22 Association of Air Medical Services (AAMS) - 20, 23, 24, 27, 72

Automatic Direction Finder (ADF) - 34

B

C

D

E

F

G

H

M

Maryland State Police Aviation Division - 83

MASH – 81

medical control -87

medical direction – 87

medical director - 86

Messerschmitt-Bolkow-Blohm - 13, 15, 17

Mobile Army Surgical Hospital (MASH) - 12, 51, 81

N

National Association of Air Communication Specialists (NAACS) – 23

National EMS Physician Association (NAEMSP) - 23

National EMS Pilots Association (NEMSPA) 23

National Flight Nurses Association (NFNA) 23

National Highway Traffic Safety Administration (NHTSA) - 80, 92

National Traffic and Motor Vehicle Safety Act - 80, 94

National Transportation Safety Board (NTSB) - 15, 16, 18, 19, 20, 21, 25, 26

Night Vision Imaging Systems (NVIS) - 26, 73

Night Vision Goggles (NVG's) - 24, 25, 26

Northeast Air Alliance (NEAA) – 89

O

P

R

S

GLOSSARY

ACCIDENT

An occurrence associated with the operation of an air ambulance that takes place between the time any person boards the air ambulance with the intention of flight/transport and all such persons have disembarked, and which any person suffers death or serious injury, or in which the ambulance was substantially damaged. This includes missions with a patient on board as well as missions that support the transport service's operations such as maintenance, training, fueling and marketing the aircraft or ambulance dedicated to the transport service.

ACLS

Refers to the Advanced Cardiac Life Support course; a syllabus and certification of the American Heart Association (AHA).

ADD-ON EQUIPMENT

Any piece of equipment that is carried onto the aircraft that is not certified by the FAA as installed equipment on the aircraft.

ADM

Aeronautical decision-making. Refers to a curriculum that addresses the mental processes used by pilots and others in determining a particular course of action.

AIRCRAFT TYPE

Particular make and model of helicopter or airplane.

ALS Transport

The transport of a patient who receives care during an interfacility or scene response commensurate with the scope of practice of an EMT-Paramedic.

ALS PROVIDER

A certified provider of skills required for advanced life support.

AMBULANCE

Any vehicle used to transport a patient including rotor wing, fixed wing, ground ambulance, boat, train, etc.

AIR MEDICAL RESOURCE MANAGEMENT (AMRM)

A specific body of knowledge that focuses on communications and team building between aviation, medical, communications and management personnel and includes human factors and situational awareness training for all disciplines of an air medical transport service.

Advanced Trauma Life Support (ATLS)

A syllabus and certification offered to physicians by the American College of Surgeons.

ATP

Airline Transport Pilot. A certificate over and above private and commercial certificates requiring higher qualifications and more stringent criteria.

BEECHCRAFT T-34 Mentor

Airplane make and model.

BLS Transport

The transport of a patient who receives care during an interfacility or scene response that is commensurate with the scope of practice of an EMT-B.

BLS PROVIDER

A certified provider of skills required for basic life support.

BELL HELICOPTERS

U.S. manufacturer for several makes and models of helicopters used by the military. The UH1H (nicknamed "Huey") was widely used in Vietnam.

BTLS

Basic Trauma Life Support; a syllabus offered by the American College of Emergency Physicians to provide a standard of care for the prehospital trauma victim.

CERTIFICATE

Signifies a pilot level of competency, i.e., student, private, commercial. It can also refer to the type of service a company is qualified to provide under Federal Aviation Regulations.

CIA

Central Intelligence Agency – a civilian foreign intelligence service of the U.S. Government.

CISD

Critical Incident Stress Debriefing – A process developed to address providers' stress following a critical incident, such as the injury or death of a crewmember.

CONSORTIUM PROGRAM

A medical transport service sponsored by more than one health care facility or entity.

CONTROLLED AIR SPACE

Air space designated as continental control area, terminal control area or transition area within which some or all aircraft may be subject to air traffic control.

CPR

Cardiopulmonary resuscitation – emergency procedure of chest compressions and artificial ventilation applied to a person in cardiac arrest.

CRASH RECOVERY

Procedures involved in responding to an aircraft crash that includes extricating persons from specific types of aircraft and knowledge and location of certain components within an airframe of a specific aircraft make and model.

CRUISE

The level portion of flight between ascending and descending.

CRM

Crew Resource Management. A term sometimes used interchangeably with ADM to reference a body of knowledge that addresses human factors and a pilot's decision-making process.

CRITICAL CARE TRANSPORT

The transport of a patient from an emergency department or critical care unit (or scene, RW) who receives care commensurate with the scope of practice of a physician or registered nurse.

DEAD-STICK LANDING

Type of forced landing when an aircraft loses all its propulsive power and is forced to land.

ED

Emergency Department

ELT

Emergency locator transmitter. A radio transmitter attached to the aircraft structure that is designed to locate a downed aircraft without human action after an accident.

EMS

Emergency Medical Services.

EVENT

The result of a chain of errors or red flags that are linked together and that do not necessarily end with an undesirable result but have the potential to develop into an incident or accident. For example, an event may result in filing an FAA 135.417 Form (mechanical interruption form) or may be a low tire not reported by driver, nor checked on daily inspection, then flat tire experienced with patient on board resulting in alternate transport or significant delay for patient.

FAR

Federal Aviation Regulation.

FIXED WING

Term for airplanes

GED

General Education Development tests used as an alternative to the U.S. high school diploma.

HAA

Helicopter Air Ambulance. Term used interchangeably with Helicopter Emergency Services (HEMS).

HAZARDOUS TERRAIN

Terrain which has significant obstacles, antennas, power lines and such within three miles of the route or has minimal visual surface reference or subtle elevation changes.

HeliExpo

Tha annual international helicopter trade show and conference sponsored by the Helicopter Association International (HAI).

HELIPAD

A designated area usually with a prepared surface used for takeoff, landing or parking helicopters.

HELIPORT

An area of land, water or structure used or intended to be used for the landings and takeoffs of helicopters and includes its buildings and facilities, if any are part of the landing site.

HEMS

Helicopter Emergency Medical Services

HF radio

High frequency radio with an electromagnetic range between 3 to 30 megahertz (MHz).

HRS-3 Sikorsky

Manufactured helicopter used by the U.S. Air Force since 1950.

HUMAN PATIENT SIMULATOR

A mannequin that has electronic or mechanical means to simulate human physiologic responses to performed skills.

IFR

Instrument Flight Rules.

IMC

Instrument Meteorological Conditions.

INCIDENT

An occurrence other than an accident that affects or could affect the safety of operations.

INDEPENDENT PROGRAM

Referring to a medical transport service not sponsored by a hospital and operating under its own FAA certificate.

INSTALLED EQUIPMENT

Includes all items or systems on the aircraft at the time of certification and any items or systems subsequently added to the aircraft with FAA approval through a Supplemental Type Certificate (STC), FAA Form 8110 or Form 337 action.

INFECTION CONTROL

An approach to reducing the risk of disease transmission from patient to care provider, care provider to patient, and from the contaminated environment to care provider or patient.

INTERFACILITY TRANSPORT

Medical transport form one hospital to another hospital (usually to a higher level of care).

LEAD PILOT

The pilot in charge of a group of pilots assigned to a base or to a program.

MEDICAL PERSONNEL OR TEAM

Refers only to the patient care personnel involved in air medical or ground transport.

MEDICAL TRANSPORT SERVICE

A company or entity of a hospital or private service which provides air transportation and/or ground interfacility transportation to patients requiring medical care. This term may be used interchangeably with the term "medical transport program" throughout the document.

MIT

Massachusetts Institute of Technology.

MODALITIES

Refers to the treatment plan and equipment used for specific patient care needs.

MOUNTAINOUS TERRAIN

Terrain over which a route (or within three miles of a route) varies in elevation more than 1000 feet.

NTSB

National Transportation Safety Board – Independent U.S. government agency responsible for civil transportation accident investigation.

OH-23D and Hiller OH-23 Raven

Light military helicopter used by the military for training.

OPERATOR

The term refers to an FAA Ceritifcate Holder

OPERATIONAL RISK PROFILE

A list and description of risks that may be encountered during normal, routine operations and often include the Risk Management elements of risk analysis, evaluation, treatment, and residual risk.

OSHA

Occupational Safety and Health Administration.

OUTSOURCING FLIGHTS

Transferring a request to another service but retaining control of the coordination throughout the transport.

PHTLS

Prehospital Trauma Life Support. A syllabus offered by the American College of Surgeons to provide a standard of care for the prehospital trauma victim.

PIC

Pilot in command.

PISTON ENGINE

An internal combustion engine that uses one or more reciprocating pistons to convert pressure into a rotational motion used mostly in small airplanes.

PROGRAM PERSONNEL

Refers to all personnel involved with a medical transport service or program (i.e., pilots, drivers, mechanics, communications specialists, medical personnel, administrators, etc.).

PROVIDER

A person who provides patient care.

QUALITY MANAGEMENT

QM is a total process of continually monitoring, assessing and improving the quality of the service.

R&R

Military slang for rest and recuperation.

RAPID FUELING

Fueling an aircraft with rotors (RW) or propellers (FW) turning.

RAPID LOADING /UNLOADING

The loading or unloading of patient(s) or equipment with rotors (RW) or propellers (FW) turning.

REFERRED TRANSPORT

A transport that is turned over to another service in all aspects, including billing/receipt of revenue for the transport. No fees are collected by the referring service.

RISK

The effect of uncertainty on objectives.

RISK MANAGEMENT

Coordinated activities to direct and control an organization regarding risk; an organized approach enabling effective management of both potential threats to objectives and new opportunities.

ROTOR WING

A term for helicopters.

SCENE RESPONSE

Response to the scene of an accident such as auto, farming, leisure, or industrial accidents, for example, that involve injuries.

SENTINEL EVENT

An unexpected occurrence involving death or serious physical or psychological injury, or the risk thereof. Serious injury specifically includes loss of limb or function. The phrase "or risk thereof" includes any process variation for which a recurrence would carry a significant chance of a serious adverse outcome.

SPECIALTY CARE MISSION

The transport of a patient requiring specialty patient care by one or more professionals who can be added to the regularly scheduled medical transport team.

SPECIALTY CARE PROVIDER

A provider of specialty care, such as neonatal, pediatric, perinatal, etc.

STERILE COCKPIT

Refers to the practice of allowing no internal or external communications except for the aviation tasks at hand below certain altitudes (when the pilot needs to talk to communications or to air traffic control, for example).

SUBCONTRACTED FLIGHTS

When another service is used to supply a portion of the transport, such as the aircraft or the medical team if the service's aircraft is not available or is not appropriate, or the medical team is not available nor appropriate.

WEATHER MINIMUMS

The minimum ceiling and visibility that an aircraft can operate under FAA Visual Flight Rules.

VOA -"Violence of Action"

Military slang for sites where enemy action is possible.

VOLPAR

Make and model airplane – Volpar Turbo Beech 18 widely used by Air America.

VHF radio

Very high frequency radio with a range of 30 to 300 megahertz (MHz).

VFR

Visual flight rules.

www.ingramcontent.com/pod-product-compliance
Lightning Source LLC
Chambersburg PA
CBHW030945090426
42737CB00007B/543